THE BOOK OF
TIBETAN
MEDICINE

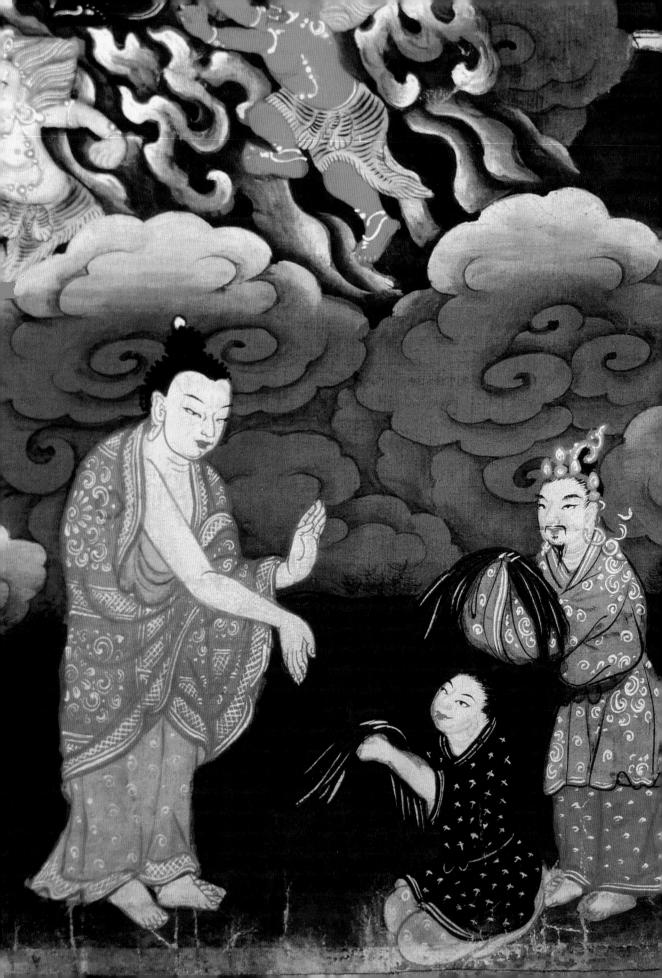

THE BOOK OF
TIBETAN
MEDICINE

How to use Tibetan healing
for personal wellbeing

RALPH QUINLAN FORDE

Any benefit you gain from this book, please attribute to my masters and all the Tibetan doctors who have ever lived. For any mistakes, please blame me.

This book is dedicated to:

His Holiness The 14th Dalai Lama, for all that you have done to protect the Tibetan people, religion, nation and this profound healing medical system from extinction. May you have a long life and realize your dreams for Tibet.

His Holiness The 17th Karmapa Trinley Thaye Dorje. May you have a long life and may your Dharma activity be successful wherever you go. May you begin once again the practice of the miraculous and precious healing pills.

The Yang Zab Dharma King.

Nicola.

Ann, who gave me the light of this life.

And healers everywhere who practise with compassion.

An Hachette Livre UK Company

First published in Great Britain in 2008 by Gaia, a division of Octopus Publishing Group Ltd
2–4 Heron Quays, London E14 4JP

www.octopusbooks.co.uk

Copyright © Ralph Quinlan Forde

Distributed in the United States and Canada by
Sterling Publishing Co., Inc.,
387 Park Avenue South,
New York, NY 10016-8810

Ralph Quinlan Forde asserts the moral right to be identified as the author of this work

ISBN: 978-1-85675-276-3

A CIP catalogue record for this book is available from the British Library.

Printed and bound in China

10 9 8 7 6 5 4 3 2 1

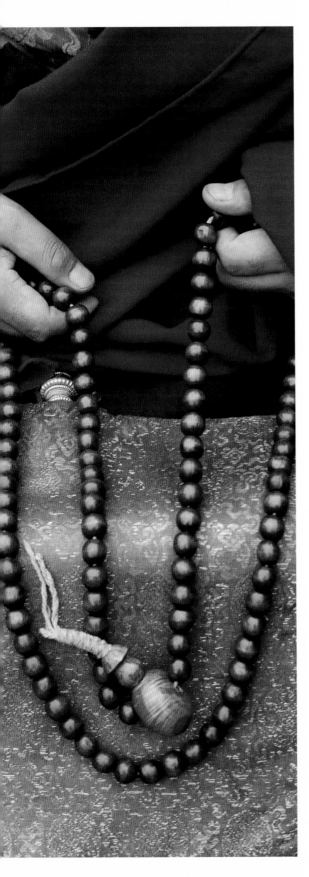

Contents

Foreword

Tibetan medicine is one of the oldest integrated medical systems in the world. This healing tradition has been practised successfully in Tibet for over 1,000 years. The science of healing — sowa rigpa — has a unique understanding of both the cause and nature of disease, the three internal vital energies and even the anatomy of 72,000 body channels as well as a vast healing pharmacopoeia. The medical tradition is based on four medical tantras *called the Gyud Zhi.*

From the time of the Buddha Shakyamuni, healing medicine and Buddhism have had a very strong affinity. This integrative system of health has treatments for both body and mind. Wherever Tibetan doctors have practised in the West, patients have remarked about their compassion.

Tibetan medicine is a very important part of Tibetan culture and by conserving and encouraging the use of the science of healing, tremendous benefits for humanity and all future generations are assured.

May all those who come into contact with Tibetan medicine have their lives protected, their diseases of pain and suffering healed and their mental anguish alleviated, and may they realize wisdom and compassion.

H.H. The 17th Karmapa Trinley Thaye Dorje

Introduction

Tibetan medicine is an ancient and profound system of healing that has been practised since the 8th century CE. The entire system, with its methods and treatments, is contained within four medical texts or tantras, known as the Gyud Zhi, which is considered by adepts of Tibetan Buddhism to be celestial in origin and therefore profoundly sacred. These ancient texts describe a medical system that integrates spiritual life into physical wellbeing and strives for the liberation of body, mind and spirit.

Specialists in all specialities

The methods of healing that are found in Tibetan medicine represent the collection and distillation, over many centuries, of the best of the ancient healing practices from India, China, Persia and Greece, fused with Buddhist Tantric science, which focuses on esoteric rites and the activity of the lama. The *Gyud Zhi* describes 404 diseases and how to treat them. Of these 404 maladies, 101 can be treated through diet, herbal remedies and techniques such as acupuncture; the other 303 ailments are said to be the result of karma (the law of cause and effect, see page 43) and may be cured only when the patient engages in ritual and prayer, or when a highly skilled healing lama physician intervenes on the patient's behalf.

Practitioners of Tibetan medicine commit these ancient texts to memory in their entirety when they train to become doctors, and thereafter refer to them daily. It takes up to ten years to train as a doctor of Tibetan medicine. Much of the learning may only be revealed to a worthy initiate by a master, because Tibetan medicine is no different from Tibetan Buddhism in stressing the importance of an unbroken lineage of transmission from the enlightened founders to the present day.

After this period of study, such is the vastness of their understanding that Tibetan doctors are equipped to practise in every medical specialism, including gynaecology, nutrition, psychiatry, palliative care, geriatrics and paediatrics. A doctor of Tibetan medicine is a specialist in all specialities simultaneously.

A healing system for the world

The *Gyud Zhi* has much to teach us today, in a world that could be described as suffering from an epidemic of stress-related illness. Throughout this book you will come to understand how the ideas in Tibetan medicine about lifestyle and proper diet can be used to benefit your health and wellbeing. Some of the advice may seem simple, but the effect on your wellbeing may be profound. Rather than simply manage disease, you can come to learn how to cure your illnesses permanently and also begin a path towards enlightenment and benefiting others with the wisdom you acquire.

The principles of Tibetan medicine apply to human beings everywhere and not just to Tibetans. The Tibetan science of healing is based on knowledge of *tsog-lung*, or vital force (see page 42), and on the protection, promotion and unique understanding of the body's internal

A mandala of Avalokiteshvara, embodiment of the Buddha's compassion. Compassion is at the heart of Tibetan medicine.

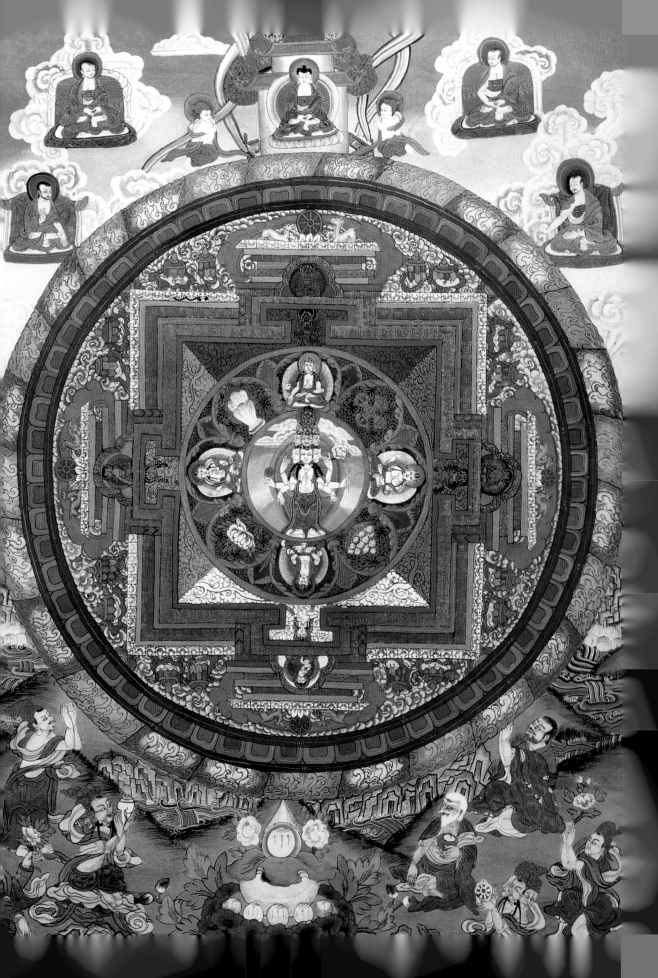

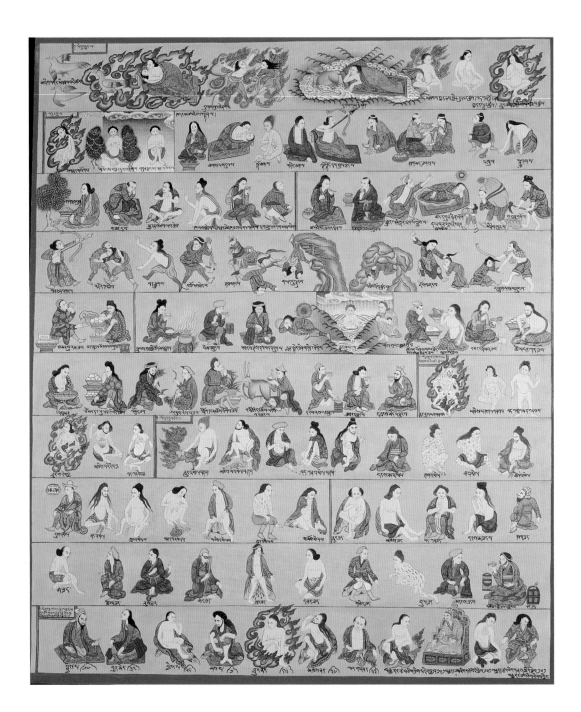

energies: *lung*, *tripa* and *bekan* (see page 50). Tibetan medicine contains the secrets of human health, homeostasis and wellbeing for everybody.

Mystical anatomy

According to the Buddhist *sutras*, or scriptures, as far back as the 5th century BCE the Buddha explained the make-up of the human body through his teachings on medicine, which are

The causes of disease, illustrated here, include bad diet and behaviour as well as the influence of the seasons and karma.

embodied in the Tibetan medicine practised today. Importantly, the Buddha saw the physical body as pervaded by an energetic body that begins at conception. While Western medicine explains that life begins with the fertilization of an egg by a sperm, the Buddha described human mystical channels. Tibetan medicine also teaches that a life force known as *la* moves around the chakras following a 28-day cycle that coordinates with the moon. On full-moon days, *la* is situated in the crown chakra and religious practice is held to be more powerful because the body's internal energies are aligned in a more spiritually potent way. Tibetan doctors always consider the position of *la* in the body before giving treatment.

Causes of disease

Tibetan medicine defines ill health primarily in terms of its cause, and then by its nature. There are four causes of disease according to the system: diet, behaviour, season and karma. For example, poor diet, negative lifestyle habits (such as smoking or overworking), seasonal changes (like excessive summer heat, winter cold or damp rains) and negative karma ripening can all cause sickness. Buddhists regard the nature of physical disease in a spiritual sense, as resulting

life as arising from the mingling of a white component from the father's semen, a red component from the mother's ovum and a blue essence called *tsog-lung*, which can be translated as 'vital force' or 'breath of life'. *Tsog-lung* controls everything in the living organism and is driven by its karmic imprint towards rebirth.

These three essences, white, red and blue, create the three main channels for mystic energy in the body. These in turn branch into a total of 72,000 minor channels that enable *tsog-lung* to pervade every part of the body (see page 48). The points at which the channels intersect are mystical energy centres that are known as chakras (see page 56).

The body's three component life forces – known respectively as *lung, tripa* and *bekan* – are believed to be held in place by the three main

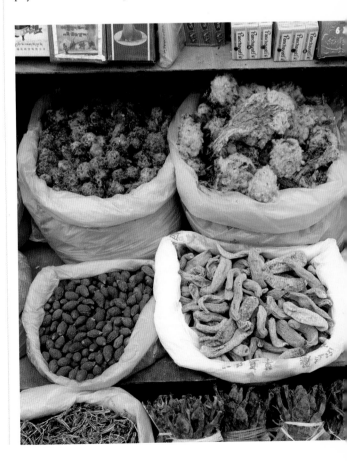

Everyday herbs and spices sold in the markets of Tibet are used in the natural remedies of Tibetan medicine.

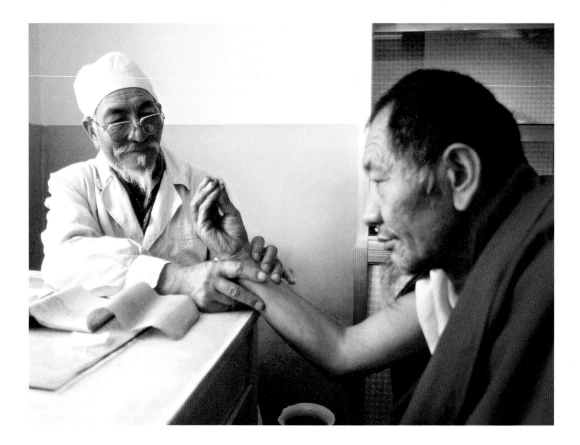

The diagnostic methods of Tibetan medicine include analysis of a patient's pulse, urine and astrological data.

from the three mind poisons – attachment, aggression and ignorance. These mind poisons throw the life forces *lung*, *tripa* and *bekan* out of balance, and the result is the manifestation of disease (see page 54).

A doctor of Tibetan medicine diagnoses which vital forces have been dislodged from their seat in the body and then sets about guiding them back into harmony. Healing in Tibetan medicine is quintessentially about using diet, lifestyle changes and, finally, therapies to return these life forces to their respective seats and thus into balance, bringing about health and vitality. Healing in this way does not simply reduce the symptoms of a condition, but benefits every part of a person, energetically as well as physically.

Lung energy is thought to be the basis of all disease because it is so closely connected to the mind and vital energy – in particular, to the subtle but profound consciousness located in the heart, known as *yi zhang ma*. Tibetan medicine teaches that energetic imbalance begins in the patient's mind as it experiences the world with a perception coloured by *marigpa*, or belief in the self (see page 54). This causes an imbalance in *lung* energy that brings about an energetic and physiological stress that pulls the other two life energies, *tripa* and *bekan*, out of harmony. Understanding the role of *lung* imbalance enables doctors effectively to treat the stress-related disorders, from depression and anxiety to insomnia and digestive problems, that affect an increasing proportion of people in the West.

The healing environment

Tibetan medicine stresses the importance of our environment to good health. For centuries, this system of healing was practised in an unpolluted homeland filled with healing herbs and pure food and water. The Medicine Buddha is often depicted in the centre of such a healing paradise, where every natural material, from rocks to plants, can be used as medicine. Tibetan medicine teaches that five elements – earth, water, fire, air and space – pervade the cosmos and make up every part of our world, including ourselves. In an unpolluted environment, these five elements are in synergy and natural items can be utilized to maintain health. A crystal is believed to combine the five elements to maximum effect, and thus impart a powerful effect within the body to restore equilibrium, since it takes a single year to create a plant, but up to 1,000 years to form just one crystal.

Diagnosing ailments

Tibetan medicine uses complex methods of diagnosis that derive from an analysis of a patient's pulse, urine and astrological data. Tibetan doctors are renowned for their ability to read pulses (see page 66). After taking three pulses on each wrist, a trained Tibetan doctor can interpret the data to understand everything that is happening within the body. The most experienced doctors supplement pulse-reading with an extra-sensory perception that has astonished Western colleagues and patients.

Urine analysis (see page 70) is another method of diagnosis, urine being regarded as a mirror of the changes taking place in the body. A doctor will also look at the patient's tongue (see page 72), as well as analysing astrological data (see page 74) to determine the lunar cycle of *la* life force, the best time to begin treatment and the origin of some psychiatric illnesses.

The tools of Tibetan healing

In Tibetan medicine, diet plays a major role in the prevention and cure of disease. The *Gyud Zhi* classifies foods according to their benefit to the three life forces, *lung*, *tripa* and *bekan* (see page 92). The text also describes the seven bodily constituents that are considered essential for life and health: saliva, blood, bone, marrow, flesh, fat and reproductive essence. These are derived from the digestive process.

Lifestyle advice, such as eating the right food for the time of year (see page 96), is an key tool in Tibetan medicine. Therapeutic intervention is always secondary to suggested changes in diet and lifestyle. In this book you will learn how diet plays a vital role in health, how management of the three energies of the body creates physical and mental wellbeing, and how the healing herbs provided by nature can contribute to a long life free from disease.

Therapies employed by Tibetan doctors include moxibustion, the burning of herbal cones on acupuncture points (see page 118); cupping, in which cups are used to create a vacuum on the patient's skin and break up accumulated toxins (see page 119); and more than 2,000 herbal formulas (see pages 102) to pacify or eliminate energies and bring the body's vital forces back into balance. Most profound of the healing tools available to the Tibetan doctor are the alchemical remedies, in particular the Precious Jewel Pills (see page 121), which contain substances such as diamond and gold and are made according to ancient rituals that last 40 days and nights.

Path to enlightenment

The fundamental aim of Tibetan medicine is not simply homeostasis – mental and physical harmony – but the spiritual enlightenment of both patient and practitioner. Meditation practice (see page 128) is highly valued as a healing tool, since all Buddhism, but especially Tibetan Buddhism, has a profound understanding of the mind and inner consciousness. To practitioners, the seat of the mind is in the heart, not the brain. The heart pervades the body energetically, creating wellbeing by balancing the three life-force energies. Practices such as meditation and yoga open up the *marigpa*, or reactive self, which antagonizes *lung* energy.

A special form of Tibetan yoga known as yantra yoga (see page 140) is also used to harmonize the three energies in the body and clear blocks in the energy channels, allowing life energy to flow freely around the body. Yantra yoga should not be practised by the uninitiated without the help of a guru, but simple prostrations (see page 138) may easily be performed at home and can also open up these blockages, enabling energy to flow freely. Smoking is thought to block energy channels and is discouraged in both Tibetan medicine and Buddhism.

The most revered healing method in Tibetan medicine is compassion, or *bodhicitta* (see page 154). *Bodhi* means 'enlightened' and *citta* means 'heart'. Most people who visit a Tibetan doctor comment on the kindness, compassion and sensitivity of the practitioner. The Tibetan diaspora believe that a doctor who practises with strong compassion has greater healing results than one who simply uses herbs or therapies as a neutral medical tool. Compassion is the key to opening and understanding the practice of healing known as *sowa rigpa*, which is not only a science, but an art, a philosophy and a way of living enhanced by spiritual principles. By such means doctors of Tibetan medicine work to bring about long-lasting cures, remissions and mental and physical balance, and in some cases perhaps also complete enlightenment.

Tibetan medicine today

The Chinese army invaded Tibet in 1950. In 1959, after the crushing of the Tibetan resistance movement, the Dalai Lama and many thousands of Tibetans fled to India, where the seat of the Tibetan government in exile is now based, in Dharamsala. To help in the conservation of Tibet's culture, the government founded the Mentseekhang, an institute of medicine that has made great strides in preserving the Tibetan medical canon, producing its own remedies and training doctors. The institute now has more than 40 branches throughout India and Nepal, and has begun scientific investigation into traditional Tibetan herbal medicines.

A number of Tibetan doctors have begun to practise in the West, and the prestige accorded to the system stems largely from the patients they have successfully treated as well as the striking lack of side-effects of Tibetan herbal formulas. If its ancient legacy is to be preserved, Tibetan medicine has to be practised as a living tradition, and all those interested in Tibetan Buddhism and meditation are urged to seek a consultation with a doctor who has graduated from one of these teaching centres in India.

'The most revered healing method in Tibetan medicine is compassion'

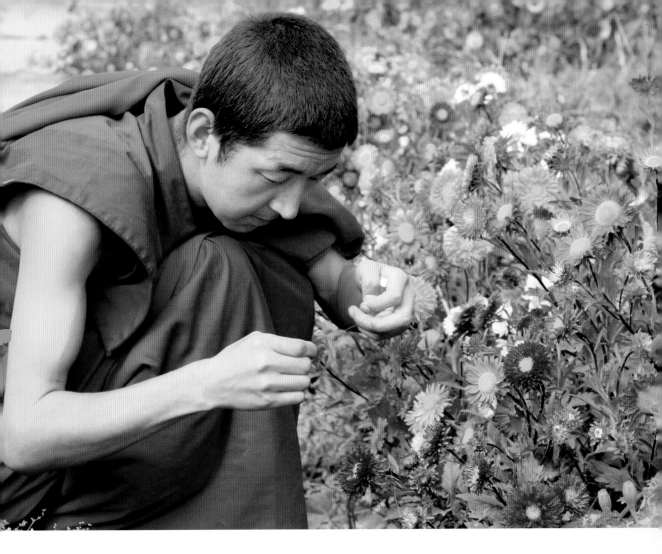

New opportunities

Tibetan medicine has an important role to play in modern medicine. Padmasambhava (see page 26), also known as Guru Rinpoche, the founder of Tibetan Buddhism in the 8th century, was a great practitioner of Tantric medicine and predicted many diseases of our age, such as cancer, AIDS and illness caused by pollution, and described special treatments for them. One of the main principles of Tibetan medicine, the importance of balancing the three energies, *lung, tripa* and *bekan*, is ignored by modern medicine, but the harmony of these energies is vital for good health.

Increasing investigation by Western science is offering opportunities for the preservation of Tibetan medicine and culture, as well as new ways to treat diseases that afflict the modern world, including diabetes, heart disease, cancer, HIV and AIDS. Promising results achieved for

Tibetan Buddhists revere the natural environment and seek to exist in harmony with all living things.

sufferers of cancer, HIV and AIDS, for example, have been reported by leading Tibetan doctors Lama Yeshe and Lama Zopa, while Dr Yeshi Dhonden, another pioneer, has completed a number of clinical trials with Tibetan herbal formulas, particularly in the treatment of breast cancer. Another exciting possibility is the development of joint ventures between Western pharmaceutical companies and the Tibetan government in exile, in order to patent and license synergistic herbal formulas. Such collaboration would provide revenue to develop Tibetan medical institutes, preserve ancient texts, conserve native plants and supply the impoverished community in exile with herbal medicines free of charge.

Another crucial contribution that Tibetan medicine can make to Western medicine is in the area of psychiatry, as this ancient healing tradition has always studied and understood the mind at a profound level. Buddhist ethics also have a valuable bearing on controversial areas of contemporary research, such as stem-cell science, in terms of encouraging a reduction of the use of animals. Buddhism also has much to offer in the area of palliative care, as it has profound practices to help the transition from this world to the next. Above all, Tibetan medicine can demonstrate to Western doctors a compassionate model of healing that promotes overall health rather than treating disease, and which urges doctors to consider the effects of treatment not only on the current lives of their patients but on all their future lives.

A universal holistic medicine

Interest in Tibetan Buddhism has proliferated in the West over the past few decades, and today it is practised in Tibet, China, India, Australia, New Zealand, Canada and increasingly also in Europe and the United States. The more people learn about its principles, the more Tibetan medicine influences the practice of medicine worldwide and helps to eradicate disease and suffering, be it physical, mental or spiritual. Genuine spiritual practice is no longer the luxury of an elite group of people, but essential for good health in a world suffering from an epidemic of stress-related ailments. Today, we crave a holistic and altruistic model of medicine that can prevent the causes of disease and heal its symptoms, while increasing wellbeing in every part of the universe. Tibetan medicine is that system.

About this book

You may not have access to a qualified doctor of Tibetan medicine, but there are many ways in which you can bring its principles into your life. The following pages outline the measures you can take to improve your health, from eating in accordance to your constitutional type to embarking on a voyage of spiritual self-discovery through practices such as yoga and meditation and the use of Buddhist ritual and prayer.

Chapter One examines the origins of Tibetan medicine and the creation of a mystical healing art. Chapter Two looks at the spiritual and medical framework of Tibetan medicine. This chapter explores how Tibetan doctors view the body's anatomy and understand disease, and explains concepts such as the three energies, vital force and the chakra system.

Chapter Three profiles the key diagnostic techniques used by Tibetan doctors, from pulse and urine analysis to tongue diagnosis and astrological divination. Chapter Four examines in depth the important role of diet in Tibetan medicine and shows how the underlying principles of this healing system can be adopted in a modern, Western lifestyle, for example by adapting your diet to your constitutional type and the rhythms of the seasons.

Chapter Five outlines key healing therapies, including the use of moxibustion and cupping and the prescribing of therapeutic herbs and the famed Precious Jewel Pills. Herbal formulas are the first remedies to which doctors of Tibetan medicine turn to restore balance to the three life energies and a range of ways are suggested in which you can use herbs and spices from the Tibetan pharmacopoeia. There's also a five-day rejuvenation programme to soothe those suffering from stress and 'burnout'.

Chapter Six examines the vital role of the mind in physical health, especially the use of meditation and yoga in Tibetan medicine. Some of these profound spiritual practices should not be attempted without a master, but everyone may cultivate compassion, bringing love and healing into their lives and the lives of others.

The final chapter discusses the central role of ritual and prayer and provides a liturgy of the Medicine Buddha, with mantras and prayers that may be used at different times.

May all sickness be healed and may *bodhicitta* grow everywhere.

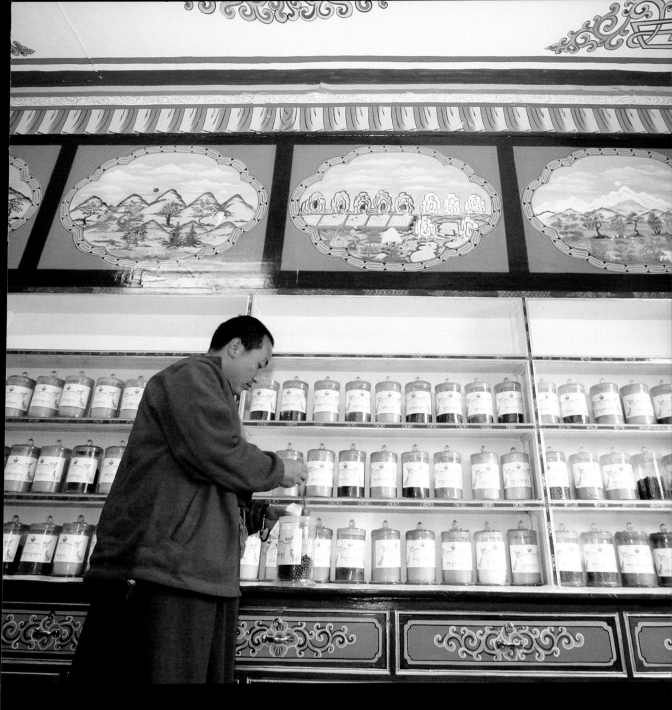

A pharmacist picks herbal remedies
according to prescription at the
Tibetan medicine hospital of

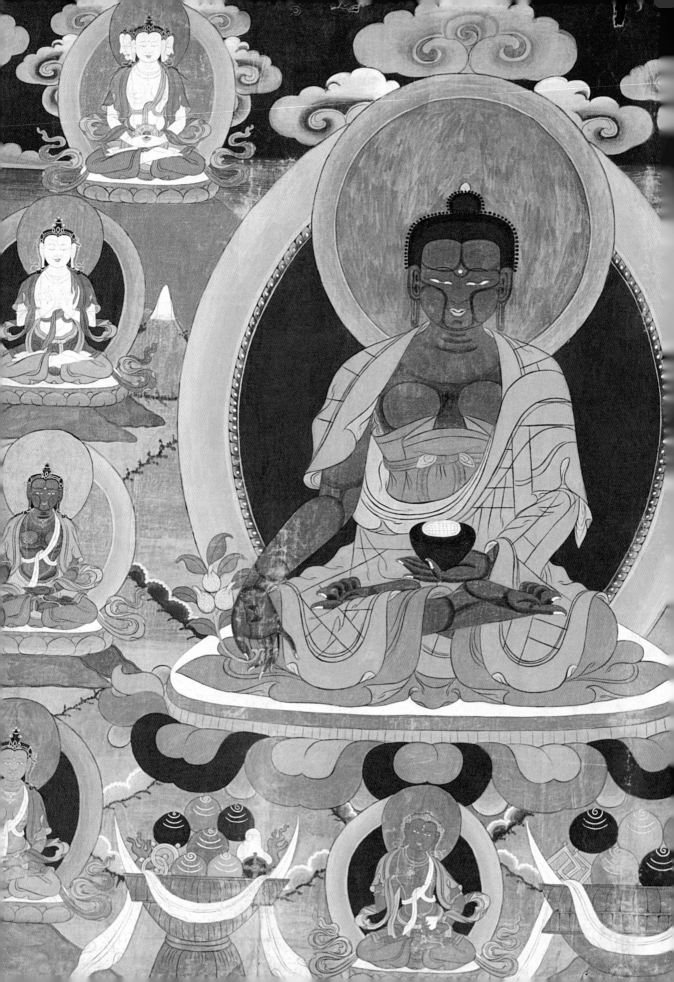

The origins of Tibetan medicine

Tibetan medicine has been renowned as a healing art since the 8th century CE. In this holistic system of compassionate medicine, the art of healing is guided by spiritual ethics and applied by contemplative sages, just as healing was once administered in cultures right across the world. Drawing its theory and techniques from ancient India, China, Persia and Greece, Tibetan medicine was fused with Buddhist Tantric science to create an unsurpassable mystical healing art that is still practised today, and from which modern Western medicine can absorb much wisdom.

Vedic mystery and medicine

The oldest information on healing within Tibetan medicine dates from the Vedic period in India (around 2,000 BCE). The sages of that culture treated not just the physical body, but also the psychic body: the part, long forgotten by modern medicine, that is thought to contain a person's life force. As in Tibetan medicine, Vedic sages taught that a person's life force flows through 72,000 mystic nerves in the body. In this way they took into account a patient's mental as well as physical wellbeing.

The Vedic Brahman caste were priests who performed religious rites, but they also became physicians of Ayurveda, the traditional healing art of India, probably because of their study and practice of spiritual texts. These texts, which set out methods of healing, disease-prevention, longevity and surgery, were thought to be the result of divine revelation, handed down orally until they were transcribed into book form alongside other aspects of life and spirituality. Thus sage-physician-surgeons evolved who were not only at the same level of enlightenment as the deeply devoted *rishis*, holy sages or seers, but perhaps at an even higher plane. They regarded health as an integral part of spiritual life and development.

The origins of medicine

According to Vedic legend, there was in the past a golden age during which human beings were enlightened. One day, the force of karma caused a man to eat a piece of bitumen. Shortly afterwards, the man developed stomach pains and started crying. The deity Brahma heard his cry, was motivated by compassion to help him and remembered the contents of the medical text taught to him by the Buddha Shakyathubcha. This Buddha, he remembered, had told him that boiled water cured digestive problems. Brahma prescribed this very remedy and it cured the man, making Brahma the first medical doctor in the history of the world.

The *devas*, or angels, then asked Brahma to teach them how they could avoid untimely death. Brahma composed 100,000 verses relating to medicine, based on the medical teachings he had received from the Buddha Kasyapa, and taught them to the *devas*. These teachings are believed to have been passed down by the *devas* to the *rishis*, who in turn passed them to the King of Benares, who was the first person in this world to receive them.

'The Vedic sages regarded health as an integral part of spiritual life'

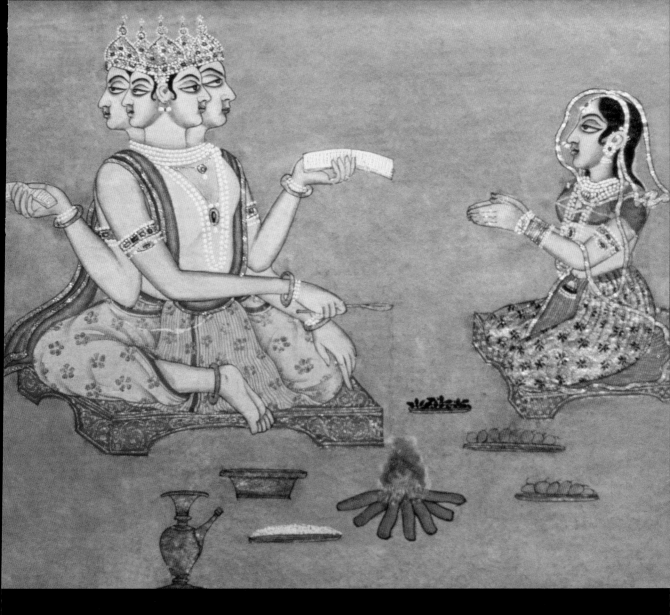

Brahma, who prescribed a remedy
taught him by the Buddha, has a
claim to be considered the world's first
medical doctor. He is shown here
holding a page from the Vedas.

The first doctor

During the 5th century BCE when the Vedic culture of spiritual healing was
flourishing, Shakyamuni Buddha (c. 563–c. 483 BCE) was born to a royal
family. Originally known as Prince Siddhartha Gautama, he abandoned
his palace and family to search for the cure that would end man's suffering.
The first human suffering he saw was disease, in the form of leprosy. Some
commentators attribute the stimulus for his quest for enlightenment
(eradicating disease from the world) to this encounter.

At the time in which the Buddha lived there were four existential medical questions: What is the disease? What is the cause of the disease? What is the cure for the disease? And how do you practise that cure? The Buddha's answers to the four questions were: egocentricity, attachment, selflessness and detachment. From these answers it is believed that Shakyamuni Buddha developed the Four Noble Truths of Buddhism: the Truth of Suffering, which states that suffering is universal; the Origin of Suffering, which decrees the cause of suffering to be craving, or selfish desire; the Elimination of that Suffering, being the elimination of craving; and finally, the Noble Eightfold Path, the technique by which one achieves the elimination of craving.

Shakyamuni Buddha is believed to have lived for four years in the Medicine Jungle, full of medicinal herbs and plants. Here, he became the Medicine Buddha and entered *samadhi*, or the state of realization, that expels the 404 diseases described in the medical treatises of Tibetan medicine. Legend tells how healing rays that were emitted from his chest in all directions drove all diseases back into space. After the rays had pervaded the entire universe, they returned to their source. Then the Buddha manifested Rigpa Yeshe, an emanation of the Medicine Buddha's mind, who announced:

The Eightfold Path

This is the means by which, the Buddha stated, one should live in order to eliminate the cravings or selfish desires, that are the cause of all suffering. The elements of the path are perfect understanding, perfect thought, perfect speech, perfect action, perfect livelihood, perfect effort, perfect mindfulness and perfect concentration.

'Because health is of the first importance,
In any undertaking, all those who want
   to meditate
And reach nirvana and who want wealth
   and happiness
Ought to learn the science of medicine.'
(Quoted in *Tibetan Medicine*, Rechung Rinpoche)

At this moment, lights emanated from the Medicine Buddha's tongue, which generated Lord Yidlas Skyes, a speech emanation of the Medicine Buddha, who asked Rigpa Yeshe to teach medicine to all those assembled. Rigpa Yeshe then taught them, through a question-and-answer session, the four *tantras* of the *Gyud Zhi,* which is translated as *The Ambrosia Heart Tantra:*

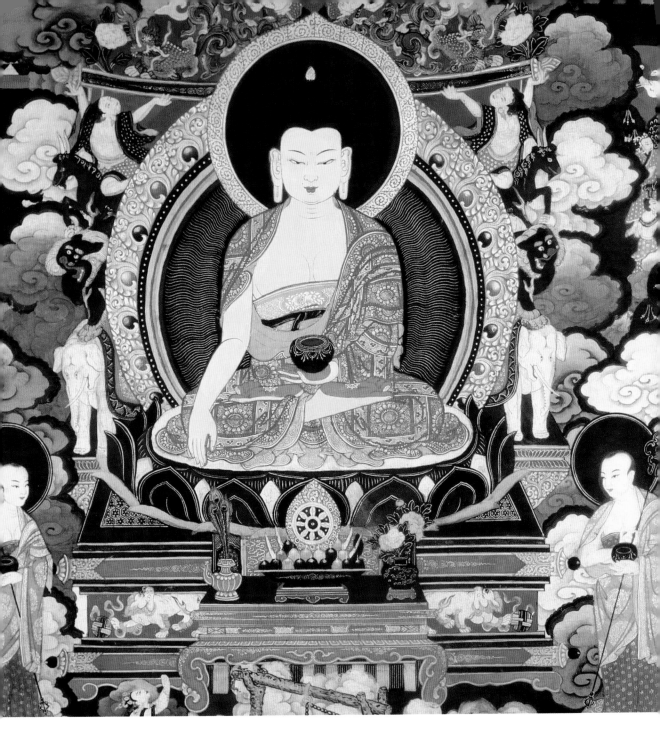

Shakyamuni Buddha taught that human disease may be cured through selflessness and detachment.

The Secret Oral Teaching of the Science of Healing. These four *tantras* are still memorized by doctors of Tibetan medicine today and referred to daily in the treatment of patients.

It is said that, due to their different karmas, the beings gathered for the exposition heard the teachings in different ways. The *devas* heard them as the *100,000 Slokas of Medicine* and the Hindus heard the *Maha Deva Treatise*. The *Gyud Zhi* was only understood completely by Lord Yidlas Skyes, who wrote down the 5,900 medical verses with lapis-lazuli ink on sheets of gold. These texts were kept in the palace of the *dakinis* (female deities) in the kingdom of Uddiyana (now in Pakistan).

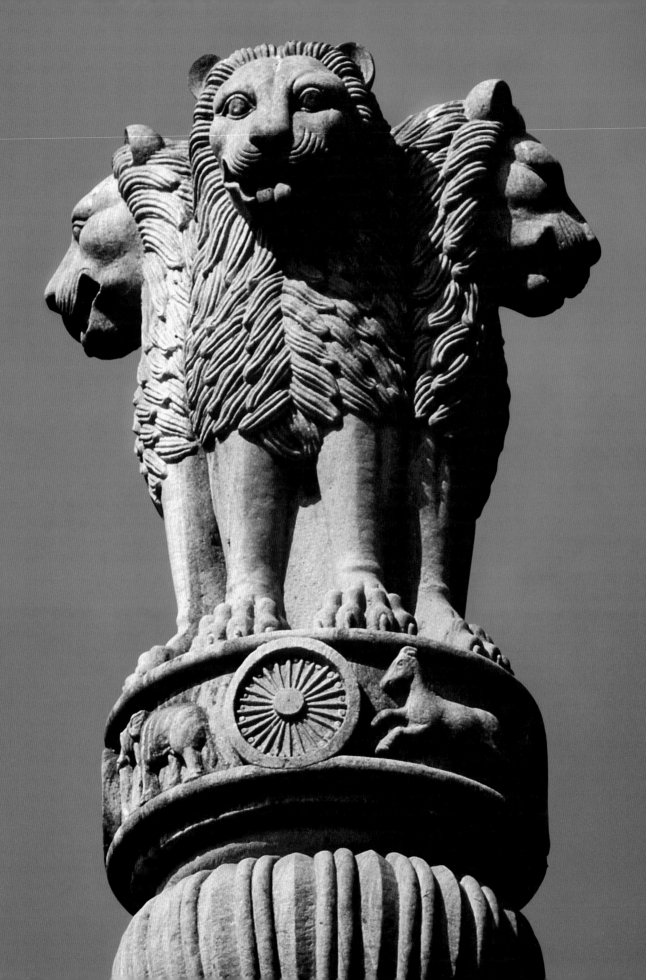

The path of the Buddha

Buddha Dharma, or the Path of the Buddha, took root in India, suffusing the Vedic healing arts with the Buddha's genius of compassion. Medicine flourished in a Buddhist environment, perhaps because the absence of a caste system within Buddhism may have opened up its practice to a wider segment of society (until that time, the study of medicine had been restricted to the Brahman caste).

Selfless service

As Buddhism spread, particularly the Mahayana form (which seceded from Theravada Buddhism in the 1st century CE), so did the healing art of compassion. This became renowned as Buddhist medicine, as its practitioners were increasingly influenced by ideals of selflessness and healed their patients' diseases. A major component of Mahayana Buddhism (as opposed to Theravada Buddhism) is the path of the *bodhisattva*. *Bodhi* means 'enlightened' and *sattva* means 'essence', and so the word describes someone whose very nature is enlightenment. Those who choose the spiritual path of becoming a *bodhisattva* pledge to postpone their own enlightenment until all sentient beings are free from suffering. In effect, they attain wisdom and compassion for the benefit of others. The Buddhist scholar Shantideva (*c.* 650–750) exemplified this path in his *Bodhicharyavatara*, a manual on *bodhisattva* behaviour that is still widely read, studied and revered by Buddhists the world over. Such ideals of selfless devotion were to have great influence on Buddhist theories of medicine.

Enlightened monarchs

Two hundred years after the Buddha passed away, the ruler of the ancient Indian Mauryan Empire, Ashoka (*c.* 269–232 BCE), converted to Buddhism

The famous Ashoka lion capital from Sarnath, India, the deer park where the Buddha first taught the Dharma.

'The art of healing pervaded every part of Ashoka's empire'

and began his remarkable and famous reign of humanitarianism. Ashoka repudiated military aggression and instead resolved to live according to Buddha *Dharma*. He established hospitals for humans and animals and promoted the cultivation of medicinal herbs. The art of healing pervaded every part of his empire, which grew to extend from present-day Afghanistan in the north to the island of Ceylon (today's Sri Lanka) in the south, and as far as the borders of Greece to the west. Throughout his lands he instigated the construction of thousands of monasteries and Buddhist shrines.

A spiritual successor to Ashoka was the 4th-century CE King of Ceylon, Buddhadasa, who also demonstrated Buddhist compassion in his promotion of medicine. He studied medicine, wrote a medical treatise and is said to have carried medical instruments with him wherever he went in order to treat his subjects, including those from untouchable castes and animals. Buddhadasa also supported village doctors and opened institutes for the care of the crippled and blind.

The transformation of Tibet

Medicine in its Buddhist form first arrived in Tibet in the 5th century CE, after two Indian Buddhist doctors saw a vision of the female Buddha Tara, who is mother of all the Buddhas. Tara told the two doctors, a man and a woman, to bring medicine to Tibet. Their work in spreading medical teachings impressed the King, Lhatho Thori Nyantsen, and he invited them to remain in his realm.

The female doctor, Vijay, married the King's son, Dungi Thorchog. He was trained by both physicians and is considered Tibet's first native lama doctor. Tibetan medicine developed within, and descended through, the Tibetan royal family.

King Songtsen Gampo

Buddhism was not formally introduced into Tibet until the middle of the 7th century, in the reign of King Songtsen Gampo (617–98 CE). He was a visionary leader and ruled Tibet at a time when it was a major power in central Asia, surrounded by Buddhist kingdoms. Historians suggest that his two Buddhist wives were the source of his inspiration to convert to Buddhism. Though one was from China and the other from Nepal, both carried Buddhist scriptures in their dowries.

By introducing Buddhism to Tibet, King Gampo not only brought medicine to the country but also sophisticated methods of rulership from China and especially from India. Although there was dissent in court over the importation of a foreign belief system and the renouncing of native shamanism, the King ordered the creation of a Tibetan script for the translation of the Buddhist scriptures, which included treatises on medicine.

He invited a number of physicians to Tibet to take part in what is considered to be the first international medical conference. It lasted for 45 years and comprised three doctors – from India, Persia (modern-day Iran) and Greece.

Individually they translated texts from their own medical systems and together they wrote *The Weapon of the Fearless One*, a medical magnum opus based on their knowledge and discussions. The Greek doctor, Galenos, remained in Tibet and established his own family medical lineage.

The first monastery

King Tritsong Detsen was enthroned in Tibet during 755 CE at the age of 13. When he was 20 years old, he invited the Bengali Buddhist Abbot Shantarakshita to come to Tibet to teach and establish Buddhism as the national way of life. The King asked him also to build the first Buddhist monastery in Tibet, but the Abbot found both the people and their protector spirits difficult to tame. Relaying his feelings to Tritsong Detsen, Abbot Shantarakshita urged him to invite the Tantric master Padmasambhava to Tibet to use his supernatural powers to subdue and transform the spirits he had encountered.

The miraculous Padmasambhava

Before his death in around 483 BCE, the Buddha predicted the birth of a Tantric adept. These predictions were recorded in *sutras* and *tantras* on no less than 19 occasions. In the *Nirvana Sutra*, for example, the Buddha tells his disciples that although his death, like the death of all living

King Tritsong Detsen, shown here, invited Padmasambhava to Tibet to establish the country's first Buddhist monastery.

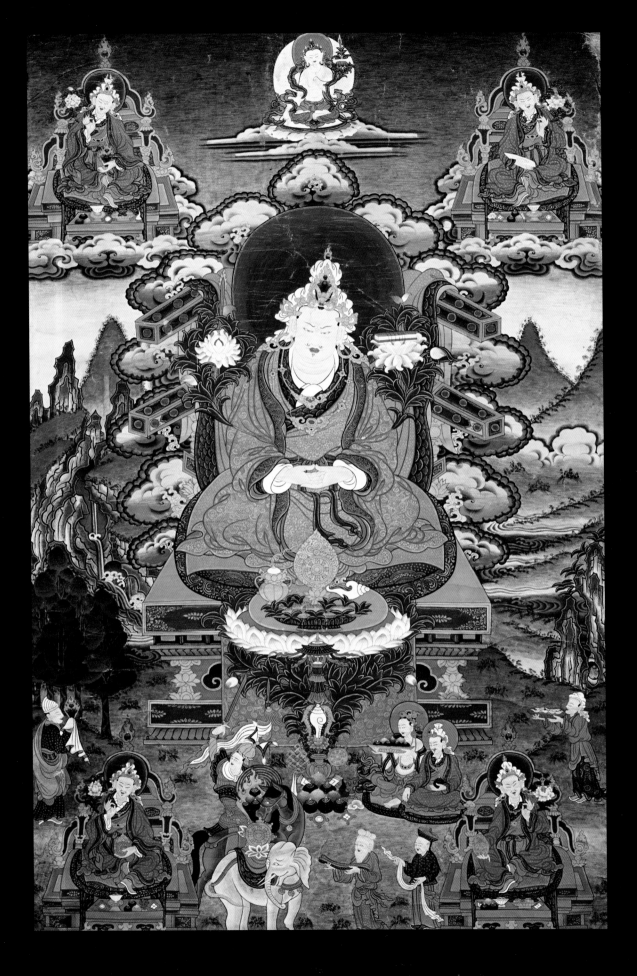

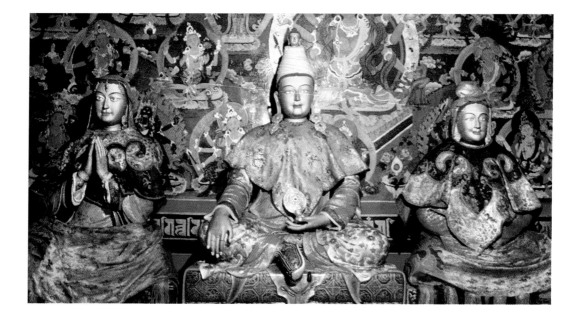

The two foreign wives of King Songtsen Gampo are said to have been the cause of his conversion to Buddhism.

things, was inevitable, they should not weep. One day, from a lotus blossom on Dhanakosha Lake in the northwestern corner of the country of Urgyan, 'there will be born one who will be much wiser and more spiritually powerful than Myself. He will be called Padmasambhava, and by him the Esoteric Doctrine will be established'.

As the Buddha had predicted, Padmasambhava was born from a lotus, in Uddiyana (today's Pakistan). He was discovered by King Indrabhuti. The King, who was a Buddhist, was journeying in search of a special jewel with which he could replenish the royal treasury, which he had emptied by making offerings to the Three Jewels (the Buddha, *Dharma* and *Sangha*) and by helping the poor. When he came across the miraculous child Padmasambhava (at that time eight years of age), he asked him who he was, to which the child famously replied:

> '*My father is wisdom and my mother is voidness.*
> *My country is the country of* Dharma.
> *I am of no caste and no creed.*
> *I am sustained by perplexity;*
> *and I am here to destroy lust, anger and sloth.*'

Padmasambhava returned to the palace with Indrabhuti, where he advised him how to rule in a way that would guide beings onto a path to enlightenment. In time, he married. At the age of 30, he saw a vision of Vajrasattva (the Buddha of purification), who asked him to leave the palace so that he might benefit sentient beings in a more active way. Padmasambhava left the palace to travel through India, transforming the eight classes of beings (protectors, demons and spirits) and meditating at cemeteries. During his travels he received instruction from Buddhist *siddhas* (enlightened Tantric adepts) on medicine, astrology, Tantric science and secret mantras. In particular, he attributed his enlightenment to Guru Shri Singha (a great *mahasiddha*) from whom he received oral instruction.

It was during a retreat that Padmasambhava received King Tritsong Detsen's invitation to visit Tibet. He went immediately, where he met the King and Abbot Shantarakshita, who had recommended him. By applying Tantric force, Padmasambhava subdued the obstructive local spirits and then helped to establish the first Buddhist monastery in Tibet, Samye Ling. This was built to a sacred geometric design that symbolized the four continents and Mount Meru, the mountain at the centre of the universe.

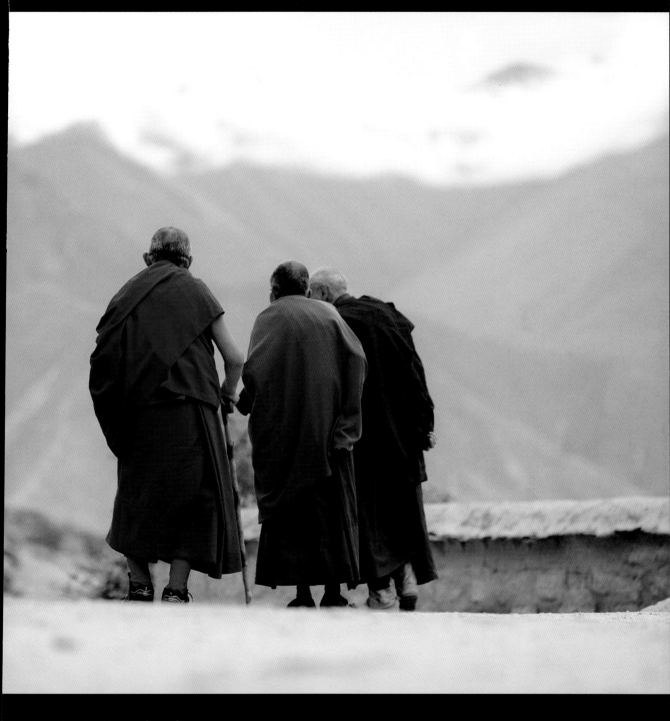

Some 1,400 years after its first introduction to Tibet, Buddhism remains at the heart of the Tibetan culture.

Guardians of the knowledge

Padmasambhava prophesied the birth of a great translator, Vairochana, and sent out a search party to find the eight-year-old child. He became one of Tibet's first Buddhist monks and a close disciple of Padmasambhava. He was educated in Tibet until the age of 15, when he was sent to India. In particular, he received teachings of the Gyud Zhi, *the four medical tantras.*

On his return to Tibet, he met Yuthog Yonton Gonpo (708–835), Tibet's first physician saint, and passed on his knowledge of the *Gyud Zhi*.

Padmasambhava instructed Vairochana to hide these sacred scriptures in a pillar of the Samye Ling monastery, to be found at a later date. Some believe Padmasambhava foresaw the destruction of monks and monasteries that would take place in the 13th century following the Muslim invasion of India, but in fact the scriptures were found by Trapa Ngonshe in 1038.

A medical conference hosted by King Tritsong Detsen, in which doctors from neighbouring regions were invited to Tibet, resulted in the translation of many more medical texts from various languages into Tibetan. From these debates, Yuthog devised the system of Tibetan medicine that has passed down in an unbroken master–student lineage to the present day.

Precious Teacher

Padmasambhava spent years in Tibet transforming its warlords and earth spirits to the path of the Buddha. He retreated to caves to undertake Tantric practices, where he left marks of his stay etched into stone, including hand- and footprints that inspired the faith of future generations of Tantric practitioners and can still be seen today. To honour his miracles and profound teachings, he became known as Guru Rinpoche, or Precious Teacher. Twenty-five of his close disciples became custodians of his secret teachings, and some of

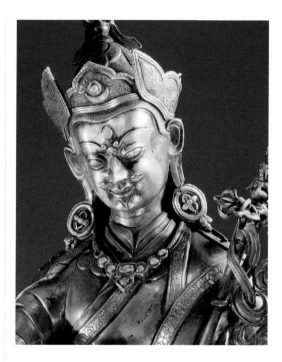

The teachings of Padmasambhava have been passed down to the present day by the lineage of his disciples.

the living embodiments of Tantric teachings come from the bloodline of Padmasambhava's original students. His hidden teachings are even today being uncovered by the *tertons*, reincarnate lamas who discover them carved into rock faces or on the ground. The *tertons* translate the healing practices that are written in the secret Dakini script, which is revealed only to close disciples and initiates of the Vajrayana system of Tibetan Buddhism.

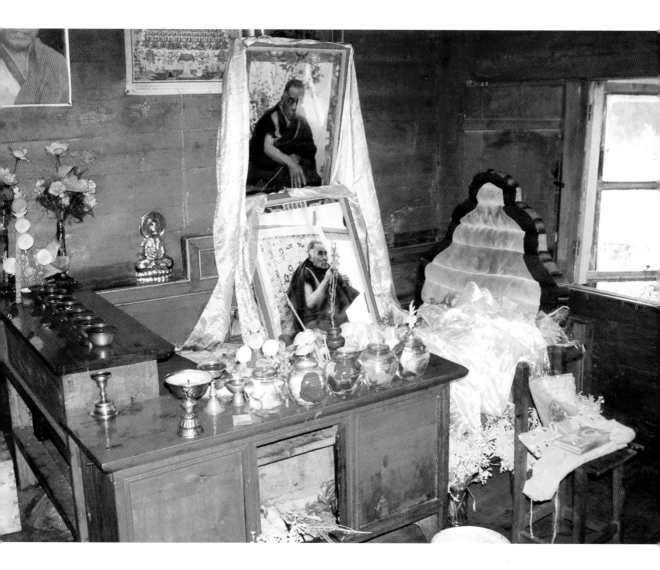

Eighty of Padmasambhava's disciples attained *jalu,* or rainbow body, in which the body dissolves into rainbow light at the time of death, leaving only hair and nails on the earth. This phenomenon is still seen today when highly realized Tantric practitioners die. A group of contemplatives from the Catholic Church have been researching the most recent case, which occurred in the summer of 1998 during the seven days after the death of Khenpo Achos, a monk from Kantze Gompa in eastern Tibet.

The tradition continues

Kunkhyen Chokyi Dragpa (1595–1659) played a crucial role in the evolution of Tibetan medicine. He was a supreme master of Tibetan Buddhism

A well-known case of jalu, *that of Khenpo Achos, occurred during 1998 in this meditation hut in eastern Tibet.*

and medicine and an adept of Tantric practice. He arranged and compiled a number of books of medicine for posterity, including, it is said, Yuthog Yonton Gonpo's medical works and the original four *Gyud Zhi tantras.* He also influenced the organization of the lineages – the unbroken chain of masters and students that reaches back to Padmasambhava. He took up leadership of the Drikung Kagyu order with his brother Konchog Rinchen (1590–1694) and held the lineage from 1626–59. This method of leadership continues to the present day through successive reincarnations.

Founding of medical schools

Fifteenth-century Tibet saw the emergence of two doctors, Jangpa (1395–1475) and Zurkarpa (1439–1475), who created rival medical systems that lasted up to the 17th century, when the influence of the sacred medicine began to decline. At this point, the great 5th Dalai Lama (1617–1682) decided to build a medical school to revive interest in the alchemical medicine of the siddhas, enlightened Tantric adepts.

Chakpori medical college

The 5th Dalai Lama asked his Regent, Sangye Gyatso, to locate a suitable site. The Regent went wandering and, when he was in the vicinity of Chakpori in Lhasa, experienced a mystical vision of a healing medicine paradise. Having received this vision, it was a simple decision to choose Chakpori as the site of the first Tibetan medical college, which was established in 1696.

It was decreed that each large monastery in Tibet would receive a doctor from this college

Established in 1696, the medical college at Chakpori was destroyed during the Chinese repression of 1959.

to serve its monks and the wider community. Tibetan medicine flourished at this centre of learning for 600 years until the Chinese repression of Tibet in 1959, when the Chakpori college was destroyed.

At the start of the 19th century, the 13th Dalai Lama (1876–1933), together with a close disciple and lama doctor, Khyenrab Norbu, who had trained at the Chakpori school, founded another medical college in Lhasa. At the age of just 33 Khyenrab Norbu saw his dream come true, when the college enrolled 150 students and produced the first Tibetan astrological calendar based on the *Kalachakra Tantra* (see page 74). They named

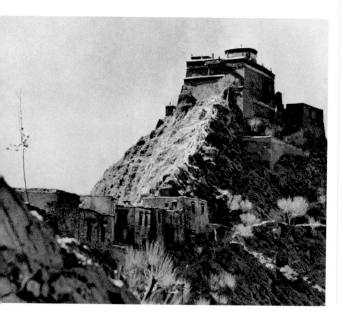

'*In the vicinity of Chakpori in Lhasa, the Regent experienced a mystical vision of a healing medicine paradise*'

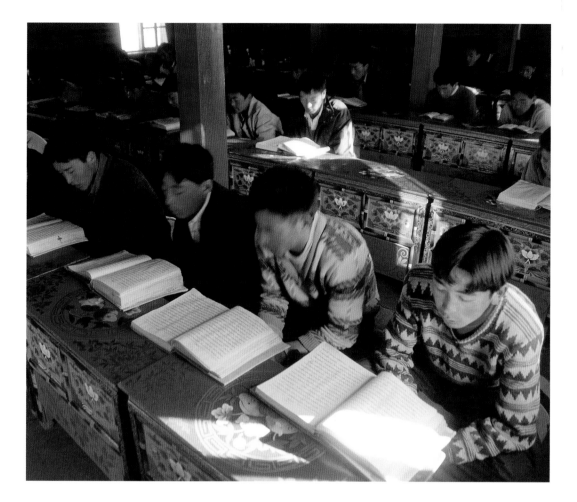

the college Mentseekhang, or the Medical and
Astrological Institute.

Threat to Tibet

In 1935, Soviet troops murdered 35,000 Buddhist
monks in Mongolia, which had converted to
Tibetan Buddhism in the 15th century as the
result of the Mongol emperor invading eastern
Tibet and coming into contact with Tibetan
Buddhist lamas. The Soviet army also destroyed
much of Tibet's religious literature and created a
new style of writing that made the spiritual
annals of Buddhist scriptures and medical texts
inaccessible. However, by good fortune *The Atlas
of Tibetan Medicine,* a collection of 76 beautiful
paintings depicting the medical system, was
saved. These works were painted in the 17th
century and it is thought that only three copies
were ever made. The volumes were rediscovered

Students at the Pelchung medical school memorize the Gyud
Zhi, *the four tantras of Tibetan medicine.*

in the late 19th century by chance and have been
republished to inspire interest in, and a better
understanding of, Tibetan medicine.

When China invaded Tibet, the Chakpori was
destroyed, along with countless monasteries and
shrines and an estimated 450,000 Tibetans (at
that time, a quarter of Tibet's population studied
peacefully and practised monastically on the path
to enlightenment). In 1995, when he was aged
six, the Panchen Lama – the second-highest lama
in the Gelupa order of Tibetan Buddhism (after
the Dalai Lama) – was kidnapped by the Chinese
government along with his family. Nobody has
seen them since. To this day, Tibet maintains its
independence and statehood, asserting that it is
under illegal occupation.

Tibetan medicine today

When His Holiness the 14th Dalai Lama (1935–) left Tibet and went into exile in 1959, he set up a new medical centre as a way to conserve and promulgate Tibet's ancient and unbroken medical system and send its doctors out into the world to teach their method. Commentators say that Tibet has been guarding its authentic healing techniques for a time when they could once again flourish, directing medicine back onto its original holistic path to benefit all humanity. Today is that time.

Leading Tibetan doctors

Just three doctors of Tibetan medicine left Tibet with the Dalai Lama, among them Dr Yeshi Dhonden. One of the first actions taken by the Dalai Lama to preserve the culture of Tibet was the establishment of the Mentseekhang Medical and Astrological Institute near the home of the Tibetan government in exile in Dharamsala

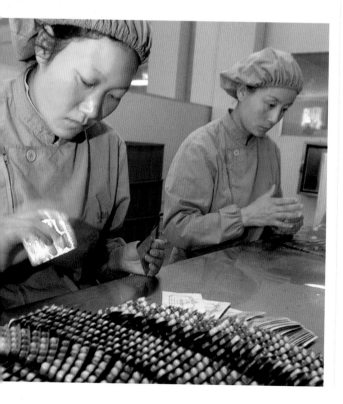

in northern India. The Dalai Lama asked Dr Dhonden to take responsibility for the running of the Mentseekhang and His Holiness personally paid for the training of Tibetan doctors at this centre. Mentseekhang-trained doctors have gone on to practise their art across the globe, including in the United States, Canada, New Zealand, Germany, Australia and elsewhere. This has been an incredibly compassionate gift to the world. Practitioners hope that in the future every medical school worldwide will teach a class on Tibetan medicine, since the best way to keep alive this ancient healing system is to study and discuss its principles and put them into practice.

Today, only around 220 practising physicians of Tibetan medicine have been trained in colleges – and only a small percentage of these serve the Western world and its huge need for healing. Among these numbers, the doctors described below are particularly remarkable.

Dr Yeshi Dhonden

Dr Dhonden stands out among all the doctors who contributed to the conservation and practice of Tibetan medicine. Born in 1929, he

The ancient Tibetan herbal remedies are now produced on an industrial scale for worldwide distribution.

Dr Lho Kunsang is renowned for his profound healing abilities and his patients have reported miraculous cures.

began his training at the age of 12 under the tutelage of Khyenrab Norbu, founder of the Mentseekhang medical institute in Lhasa. After this training, he served for more than 20 years as personal physician to the Dalai Lama.

Dr Dhonden has astounded doctors and patients across the globe with his healing abilities and natural talent for explaining the theories of Tibetan medicine to those new to the discipline. In 1995 he became involved with the University of California in the first study of Tibetan medicine in the West, in the area of breast cancer. He has written numerous books in order to preserve the practice and tradition of Tibetan medicine, and is still helping and healing up to 500 patients a week at his private clinic in India.

Dr Lho Kunsang

Auspicious signs, such as the turning of a bucket of water into milk, are said to have surrounded the birth in 1942 of Dr Lho Kunsang. When he was eight years old, the 16th Karmapa recognized him as the eighth incarnation of the Lho Konchog Trinlay Namgyal lineage, which had originated from one of the original 25 disciples of Guru Rinpoche. As part of his studies, he became one of the 25 *tulkus*, educated by the second Jamgon Kongtrul of Zhe-chen.

Dr Kunsang suffered imprisonment during the Chinese occupation of Tibet. He worked as a blacksmith, carpenter and tailor by day, while carrying on his *Dharma* practice in secret. At the time of China's Cultural Revolution, when the monasteries were under attack, he hid texts and relics to save them from destruction. The relics that he protected included a sacred statue of the Buddha, whose chest has the ability to emit a sensation of heat.

Dr Kunsang is known for his incredible healing abilities as well as for an encyclopedic medical knowledge. Patients have reported miraculous healing following treatment given by him. Today,

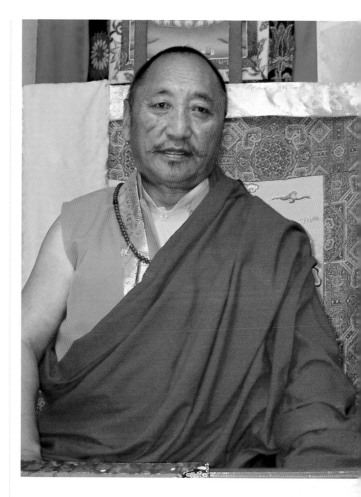

Dr Kunsang is rebuilding his monastery, Palme Gonpa, in eastern Tibet.

Dr Keyzom Bhutti

Dr Bhutti was born in Tibet to two very *Dharma*-minded parents of noble family. Her father was head of the region and her uncle was secretary to His Holiness Sakya Trinzin, head of the Sakya lineage of Tibetan Buddhism. In 1959, at the age of 12, she fled the Chinese repression of Tibet, travelling with her family to India and Dharamsala, where she was accepted to train as a doctor of Tibetan medicine.

Her training lasted for eight years under the tutelage of the Mentseekhang in exile. For three years the Dalai Lama himself paid for her tuition until a foreign sponsor was found. The conditions of refugee life were hard for this first medical class in exile, and of 15 students only six

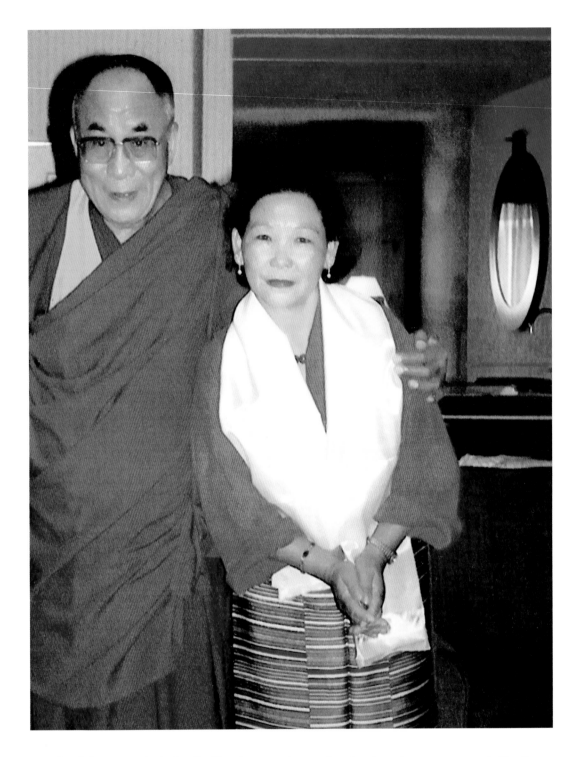

completed the course, including Dr Bhutti. After she qualified, Dr Bhutti was chosen by the Tibetan government in exile to set up a medicine clinic in Darjeeling. She now lives in Boston in the United States, where she runs a successful private practice.

One of the few Tibetan doctors operating in the West, Dr Keyzom Bhutti was sponsored by the Dalai Lama.

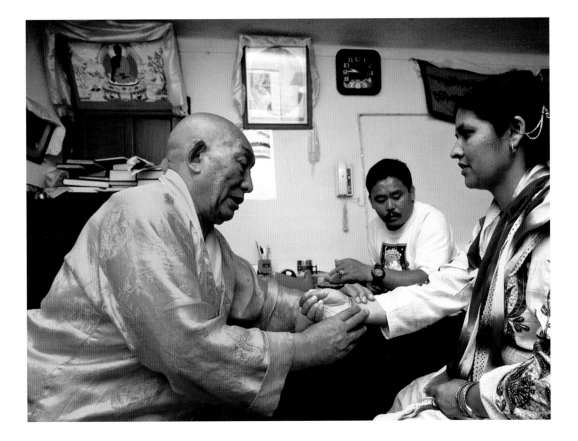

Dr Yeshi Dhonden has written extensively on Tibetan medicine to promote its dissemination worldwide.

Ven. Dr Trogawa Rinpoche

Dr Trogawa Rinpoche (1931–2005) was born into a noble family and at the age of 16 went to Lhasa to study Buddhism and medicine with the great Tibetan doctor Lhundrub Paljor, who held the lineage of the Chakpori school of medicine. Dr Trogawa practised medicine in Tibet until 1957, when he moved to Sikkim in the company of his master Jamyang Khyentse Chokyi Lodro. In 1961 he moved to Darjeeling and then to Dharamsala in 1963, to become chief medical teacher at the Mentseekhang medical institute.

In 1994 Dr Trogawa founded the Chakpori Institute of Tibetan Medicine in Darjeeling, to conserve the Tibetan medical lineage of this school, which was first established in Lhasa during the 17th century (see page 32). His students have commented that he was a spiritual master of such elegance that he was able to transmit the essence of the Buddha mind with just a word, a nuance or even a gesture.

The Chakpori Institute in India has produced 30 doctors since its inception in 1993. In 2003, the school admitted 20 female students, as Dr Trogawa intended.

The two Contreras

The best expression of the *bodhisattva* ideal in Western medicine must be Drs Francisco and Ernesto Contreras. Francisco runs the Oasis of Hope Hospital in Tijuana, Mexico, which specializes in the humane treatment of cancer patients and was founded by his late father (1915–2003). Over a period of 40 years father and son – a pathologist and surgeon – have treated more than 42,000 cancer patients using both orthodox and complementary medicine. The late Ernesto Contreras was renowned as a doctor who truly loved his patients and who pioneered the mind-body-spirit treatment of cancer.

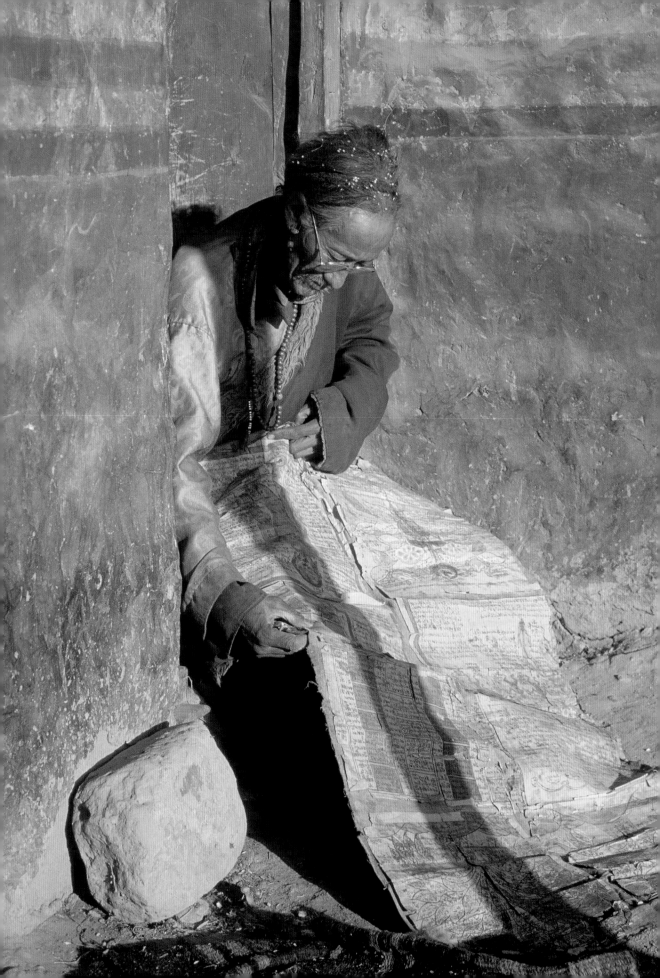

Spiritual and medical foundations

Doctors have always been revered in Tibetan culture.
Referred to by the honorific title Amchi, they are
regarded as living representations of the Medicine
Buddha and signify the long Buddhist lineage of
healing. According to the Gyud Zhi, anyone wanting
to become a doctor should possess a good intellect
since he or she will have to memorize every part of
these challenging medical tantras. Equally, potential
doctors must practise the path of the bodhisattva.
This altruistic dedication towards the liberation of
all sentient beings is in itself said to cause healing
to occur. Dualism is absent in Tibetan medicine.
Doctors and patients understand fundamentally
and experientially that mind and body are one.

The four medical *tantras*

The Gyud Zhi *or* The Ambrosia Heart Tantra: The Secret Oral Teaching of the Science of Healing *is unique to Tibetan Buddhism and, being more than 1,000 years old, forms one of the most ancient medical texts in the world. Those who wish to become doctors of Tibetan medicine must memorize its four* tantras *in their entirety – they are made up of 5,900 verses separated into 156 chapters.*

The canon of Tibetan medicine comprises more than the *Gyud Zhi*. It also includes the *Tangyur*, the Tibetan translation of the Buddha's *sutras*, and the *Kangjur*, a compendium of religious and philosophical commentaries that contains some 21 Ayurvedic medical texts but not the *Gyud Zhi*, which is classed as *terma*. *Terma* writings are Tantric spiritual texts that have been discovered at special times; they are believed to be celestial in origin and to form the basis of all medicine in the world and universe. The texts in the *Kangjur* were written by human authors influenced by Ayurvedic medicine.

The contents and their impact

Embedded in these sacred texts are elaborate descriptions of the eight branches of Tibetan medicine: general bodily health, paediatrics, gynaecology, psychiatry, wounds inflicted by weapons, toxicology, geriatrics and fertility. The knowledge contained within the texts was known to the *siddhas* before the 8th century CE and they passed it down orally.

Only the first and second *tantras* of the *Gyud Zhi* have been translated into English, but many commentaries have been written over the centuries to explain their contents, since to begin a study of these *tantras* is said to be like jumping into an ocean and requires the assistance of a qualified guide and master. One of the most famous commentaries is *Vai-dur-ya ngon-po* or *The Blue Beryl*, written in the 17th century by

---

The contents of the *Gyud Zhi*

The First *Tantra* – root – six chapters
History
Outline of all the medical *tantras*
The tree of health
The causes, diagnosis and treatment of diseases

The Second *Tantra* – explanatory – 31 chapters
Anatomy and physiology
Life cycle
Signs of death
Lifestyle and behaviour
Diet medicines

The Third *Tantra* – oral – 92 chapters
101 disorders of the three humours
Causes, symptoms and treatment

The Fourth *Tantra* – conclusive *Diamond Tantra* – 27 chapters
Urine and pulse diagnosis
Medical ingredients
Moxibustion
Golden needle therapy
Secret remedy preparations

Sangye Gyatso, Regent of the 5th Dalai Lama. It is a complete, illustrated overview of the medical system, with extensive commentaries on the four medical *tantras*.

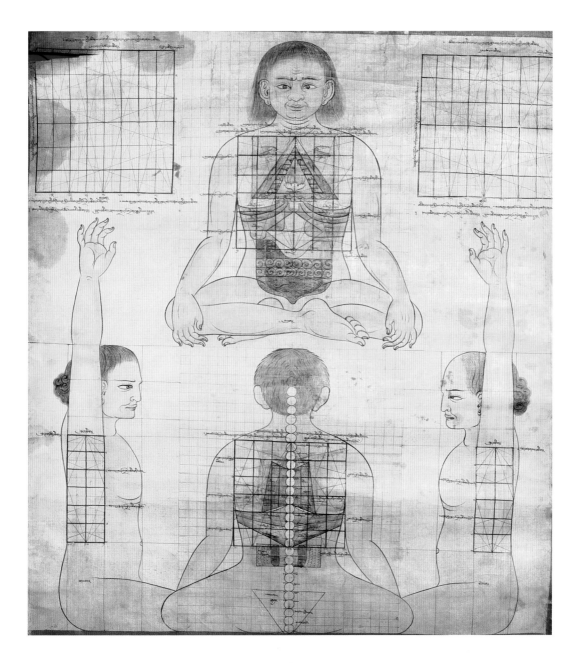

An illustration of the internal organs from The Blue Beryl, *the 17th-century commentary on the* Gyud Zhi.

In the 1960s the translation of another *terma* text, *Bardo Thodal* or *The Tibetan Book of the Dead*, became a bestseller. It was believed to have been composed by Padmasambhava and was found in the 14th century by Terton Karma Lingpa. Its publication boosted the spread of Tibetan Buddhism in the United States and elsewhere. The text is usually read out to the dying to guide them through the process of death. Study of the book, which describes the mind at the time of death, caused a paradigm shift in psychology,

culture and self-understanding. The psychoanalyst Carl Jung described the work as a parallel to psychoanalysis and said that it was often at his side. More than simply teaching aids for doctors of Tibetan medicine, such medical texts are spiritual gateways. If digested by Western medical practitioners, they could have an immense impact on the practice of modern medicine.

Vital force and divine intelligence

The central pillar of Tibetan medicine is the concept of vital force. This universal life energy, or divine intelligence, is thought to pervade the body and give life to it — without it, the body is nothing more than a shell or corpse. The more vital force we have flowing internally, the more alive we feel. In China this energy is referred to as chi *while in India it is* prana; *the ancient Greeks knew it as* pneuma *and in Tibetan it is* tsog-lung. *This concept is also specifically defined in 95 other cultures all over the world.*

For example, the Q'ero Indians of Peru have an understanding of a concept that is very similar to *tsog-lung*. They give the name *animu* to the universal life energy, the free energy of the cosmos. In *Keepers of the Ancient Knowledge*, Joan Parisi Wilcox quotes Don Americo, a shaman of the Q'ero tradition talking about *animu* in words that could equally be applied to *tsog-lung*:

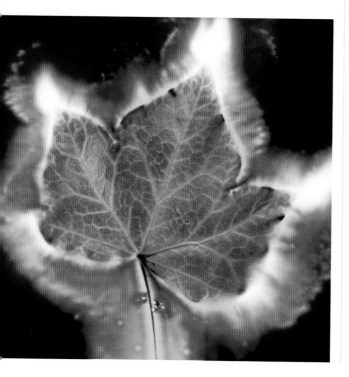

'The cosmos and everything in it is a field of energy. The stone. The star. You. Everything radiates and is penetrated by filaments of luminous energy. In any kind of situation, you have the choice of connecting with the energy that flows in the cosmos. You truly can transform that energy into love... This is the essential principle of the art of magic in the Andes.'

Kirlian photography

Vital force is the mystical consciousness that makes all the body's systems work in harmony with one another. Because life energy is beyond physical materialization, people brought up in the West may find problematic the concept that something with no form contains all forms, and that something with no definable quality encompasses all of life, touching everything from ourselves to our food and imparting vitality to it. Kirlian photography, in which an object is placed on a photographic plate and the plate is subjected to a high-voltage electrical charge, is one method of visualizing the life force. In Kirlian photographs, the energy field of a living thing may be detected as a coloured halo and has

Kirlian photography offers us a means of understanding the hidden life force that pervades us all.

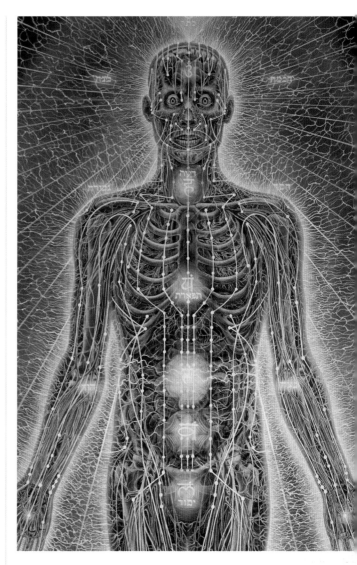

This excellent illustration of a body's energy flow also depicts the chakras of Hindu thought.

been shown to vary in brightness and colour according to the wellbeing of the subject.

The scientific evidence

Mainstream science rejects the idea of vital force because no researcher has so far been able to prove its existence using Western scientific models of investigation. However, neither have researchers been able to disprove its existence. Healers the world over, including practitioners of reiki, reflexology, acupuncture, chi gung, shiatsu, Ayurveda, shamanism, homeopathy and naturopathy, continue to use the concept of vital force as a primary method of healing disease and promoting health and happiness. These 'alternative' concepts of healing are now very popular. For example, 30 million people regularly use homeopathy in Europe, while in the United States 2.5 million Americans have made five million visits to a homeopath and spend $250 million per annum on homeopathic medicines.

Imbalances in energy flow

Tsog-lung energy flows through the body along a network of mystic channels (see page 48). When *tsog-lung* flows freely, all parts of the body and mind work as they are intended and wellbeing and freedom from disease result. However, if

there are blockages in these channels, vital force can be prevented from reaching all parts of the body. Disease is thought to set into such energy-deficient areas because Tibetan medicine regards disease as the opposite of health – and thus as the opposite of *tsog-lung*. When the flow of vital force is restored, disease is said to leave the body in the way that it entered, as the *tsog-lung* pushes out negative energy. The vibration of the body, or its energy charge, then shifts from a diseased state to a healthy, vitalized one.

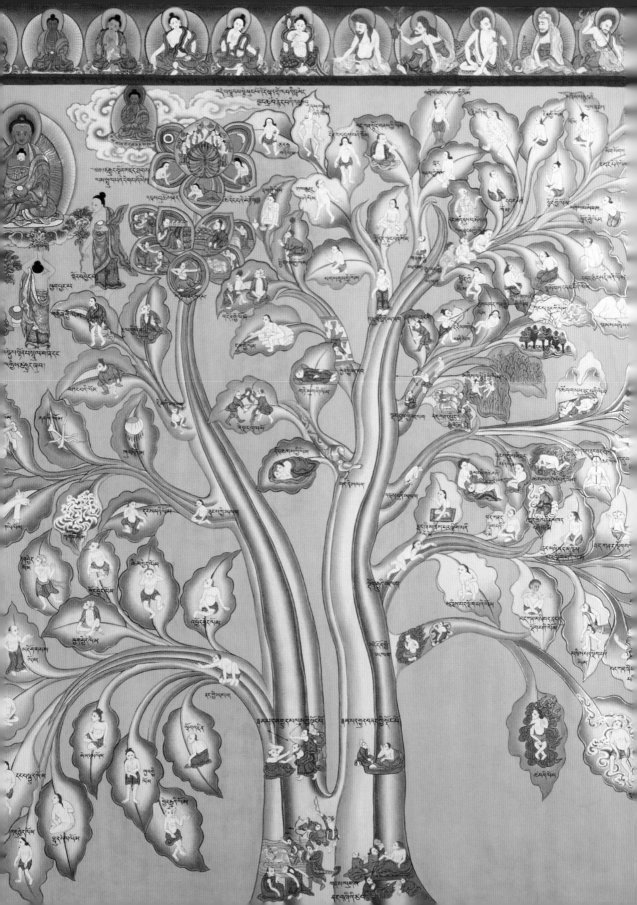

The tree of health and disease

Tibetan medicine adopts the image of a tree to help us visualize abstract notions of health and disease. Indeed, students of Tibetan medicine use this as their key tool for memorizing its many aspects. Like a mind map, the image of the tree of health and disease illustrates the whole medical system.

Understanding the image

The trunk of the tree of health and disease is in two parts. The left part of the trunk depicts health and has three branches. One represents the humours, physical constituents and excretions; the second branch shows freedom from disease and a long life; the third branch shows religious practice, wealth and happiness. The right side of the trunk depicts disease and has nine branches, representing cause, condition, entrance, location, pathways, time of arising, fatal effect, side-effects and condensation.

The lower branches of the tree stand for the three life forces known as *lung, tripa* and *bekan* (see page 50). The middle branches represent the seven bodily constituents (nutritional essence, blood, flesh, fat, bone, marrow and regenerative fluid), while the upper branches symbolize the body's three excretory functions (excrement, urine and perspiration). In order for good health to be maintained – for the tree to flourish – the three life forces, seven bodily constituents and three excretory functions must work in harmony.

The results of disease are depicted on a set of nine leaves. Negative reactions or side-effects to treatment are also depicted, to ensure that the doctor can both diagnose and treat the condition as it arises. These are caused by overdosing or insufficiently treating a particular humour. However, Tibetan medicine has a long reputation of causing few negative side-effects.

Used as a memory aid by students, the tree of health and disease depicts principles of disease prevention and cure.

Other medical images

A further two types of painting illustrate the root *tantra* of the *Gyud Zhi*: diagnosis and treatment. The medical painting of diagnosis depicts visual forms (tongue and urine), touch (pulse) and questioning. These techniques are used to build up a clear picture of an individual's bodily health.

The painting of treatment represents diet, behaviour, herbal medicine and external therapies such as moxibustion, massage and blood-letting.

By memorizing these paintings a doctor can access all the information he or she needs about health and disease and its successful treatment.

'For the tree to flourish, the three life forces, seven bodily constituents and three excretory functions must work in harmony'

Physical anatomy

Tibetan medicine has a long history of dissecting the human body and this enabled its practitioners to gain an understanding of anatomy and organ function much earlier than their Western counterparts. Tibetan doctors combine their knowledge of the physical body with an awareness of the workings of a subtle body (see page 48), which is considered in some aspects to play a more important role in healing than the physical body system.

Studying the human body

One of the guiding principles of Buddhism is that the body without its spirit, or *tsog-lung*, is no more than a corpse or empty vessel. In the past, this attitude meant that after death the body was not considered as taboo as it was in Western societies. Tibetan doctors were able to study anatomy by dissecting bodies at a time (from the 8th to the 15th centuries) when their counterparts in the West were banned from such exploration. In 1489, for example, Leonardo da Vinci began an anatomical study of the body by dissecting 30 human corpses. Pope Leo X halted his work on moral grounds, just as, so some commentators believe, Leonardo was on the verge of understanding blood circulation.

A custom of Tibetan culture that permitted the study of anatomy was *jhator*, or sky burial. In this ritual, which continues today, a corpse is brought to a mountain ledge, where it is cut to pieces and fed to the vultures as a final act of generosity on behalf of the deceased. Historians believe that such access to the body in its dismembered state explains the high level of anatomical and internal organ detail found in the paintings of the 17th-century Tibetan medical work, *The Blue Beryl*.

There are records of Tibetan paintings illustrating anatomy dating from the 13th century. Tibetan medical masters even had illustrations of the weekly developmental stages of the foetus, such was their knowledge of physical anatomy from earliest times. As far back as the 8th century Tibetan practitioners knew that the average person has 35 million skin pores and 21,000 hairs. Detailed information about the skeletal framework was also conveyed in pictorial form: 360 bones of the body were described in 23 different categories with 28 major and 210 minor joints. The medical paintings also depicted the points used for moxibustion and cupping (see pages 118–119)

The body's hierarchy

The heart is considered to be the king of the bodily kingdom and is located at the centre of the body. It is responsible for blood being transported throughout the body and also for emotional stability and mental balance. The liver is the body's queen, and the lungs are its ministers. The spleen is the governor supplying nutrients to the body. The kidneys are referred to as ministers, who manage the bodily foods. The reproductive organs (testes and ovaries) are the body's treasures, which produce the reproductive essences that in turn create the heart drop, or luminous Buddha sphere in the heart (see page 58).

Tibetan doctors early gained a profound knowledge of the human body, thanks in part to the custom of sky burial.

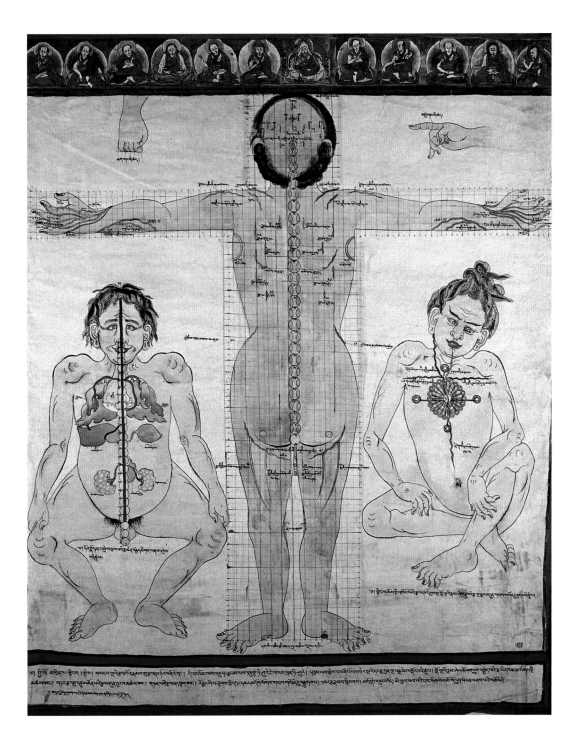

'The body without its spirit,
or tsog-lung, *is no more than*
a corpse or empty vessel'

Mystical anatomy

Although having easy access to body parts for study was important to early Tibetan doctors, it was their profound knowledge of internal Tantric anatomy that catalysed the expansion of the Tibetan healing art. The major area of study that contributes towards an understanding of Tibetan healing is an awareness of the anatomy of mystic channels known as rtsa *that transport life force around the body.*

The life-force channels

Tibetan medicine teaches that each one of us has a total of 72,000 *rtsa*, mystical channels that carry *tsog-lung* (see page 42), the breath of life, through every part of the body according to a pathway determined by the cycle of the moon. Tantric healers and practitioners consider these invisible channels to be as important as – if not more important than – the nervous and vascular systems. They are described as forming the *phra-bailus*, or subtle body, and all points for acupuncture, moxibustion, cupping and blood-letting in Tibetan medicine are based on this subtle-body anatomy.

The *rtsa* divide into three main channels: the *uma*, or central channel, where *lung* energy predominates; the *roma*, or solar channel, where *tripa* energy predominates; and the *rkyan ma*, or lunar channel, where *bekan* energy predominates. The central channel is connected to subtle life-force airs. The *roma* channel links with the blood and veins, while the *rkyan ma* channel is concerned with water and veins.

The points at which the *roma* and *rkyan ma* channels wrap around the central channel provide the location of chakras, which are the subtle body's core energy centres (see page 56). The *Gyud Zhi* is very detailed in its description of the Tibetan chakra system, stating how each chakra contains four channels that branch into 24 sub-channels, which further divide into 500 minor channels.

Blockage and disease

Each of the three main energy channels is connected to 24,000 minor channels. Tibetan medicine teaches that, if these channels remain unblocked and *tsog-lung* is allowed to pervade them as it should, health remains well balanced. However, if any of these channels become blocked, energy flow is halted and physical or mental disease results.

How life force develops

In Tibetan medicine particular emphasis is placed on the mystical power of the *tsog-lung* to start the growth of the foetus in the womb and to direct its subsequent evolution. The *Gyud Zhi* describes how, at the moment of conception, the white essence of the father's sperm and the red essence of the mother's ovum fuse with the blue essence of consciousness that represents *tsog-lung*. It is this divine intelligence that directs the formation of the physical body's organs, cells and body systems – as well as the mystical body's subtle anatomy.

During the first three weeks of life after conception, *tsog-lung* is said to develop into the life channel (*thog mar chhags-pa'i rtsa* or *srog rtsa*) that lies between the heart centre and the navel. By the ninth week in the womb all the chakras that lie in the subtle body are formed, enabling *tsog-lung* eventually to pervade the 72,000 energy channels or mystical nerves that extend throughout the human body.

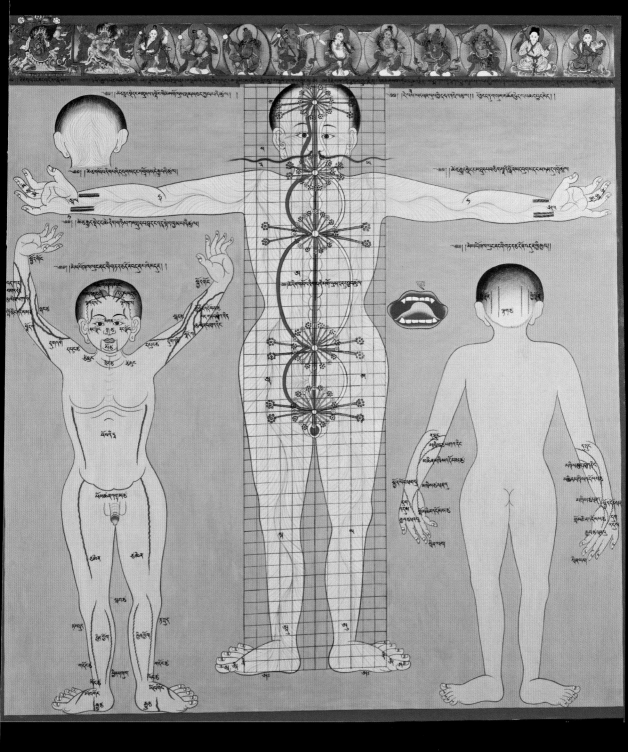

Tibetan medicine teaches that the body has a mystical as
well as physical anatomy, based around the chakras.

The three energies of health

Tibetan medicine identifies three nyepa energies that pervade the subtle body, symbolized by a bird, a snake and a pig. It is the combination of these subtle energies that dictates the individual's constitutional type and disposition. A doctor of Tibetan medicine seeks to determine which of these three vitalities predominates in the patient's make-up, then treats the patient according to his or her individual energetic constitution.

Roots of disease

According to the *Gyud Zhi*, an imbalance in the three *nyepa* energies is the very nature of ill health, giving rise to the 404 diseases. The cause of such imbalance is traced back to one of four factors: diet, behaviour, karma and season. The Buddhist notion of belief in the self (*marigpa*) also informs the Tibetan analysis of disease (see page 54).

Lung energy

This constitutional energy force is concerned with movement. It is based around the hip and genital area of the body, although *lung* is considered to be a neutral energy that mixes with the other two *nyepa* energies and so pervades every part of the body through the 72,000 mystic channels. The amount of *lung* in the body could be contained in the human bladder, state the medical writings.

Lung is thought to be the controlling force of the body, alongside the nervous system. This energy directs breathing and governs the five senses. It holds the other two energies – *tripa* and *bekan* – in balance. *Lung* energy is also responsible for the movement of blood and lymph fluids around the body.

Imbalances of *lung* are associated with diseases of the vascular system. Mental illness is caused by stress that increases the *lung* energy in the body, causing the *tsog-lung* to flow inwards and

bringing about psychosis. However, *lung* imbalance is actually involved in all disorders, since it runs through all 72,000 energy channels.

Tripa energy

The constitutional energy force known as *tripa* is concerned with metabolism and resides around the diaphragm and liver. According to the Tibetan texts, the amount of *tripa* energy in the body could be contained in the scrotum.

As a transforming force, *tripa* energy is closely associated with the element of fire. In the body it is connected particularly with the endocrine system and with the energy that is released from digestion through enzymatic processes. An excess of *tripa* leads to health conditions relating to the liver, gallbladder and small intestine.

Bekan energy

This constitutional energy force is fluid in nature and is believed to reside in the head. The amount of *bekan* energy in the body could be contained in six handfuls, according to the medical texts.

Bekan energy is responsible for lubrication and it oversees fluid levels in the body and the smooth movement of joints. *Bekan* energy is also connected to the anabolic processes that build organs, bones and muscles, and it plays

This thangka illustrates how the three energies combine to create different constitutional types.

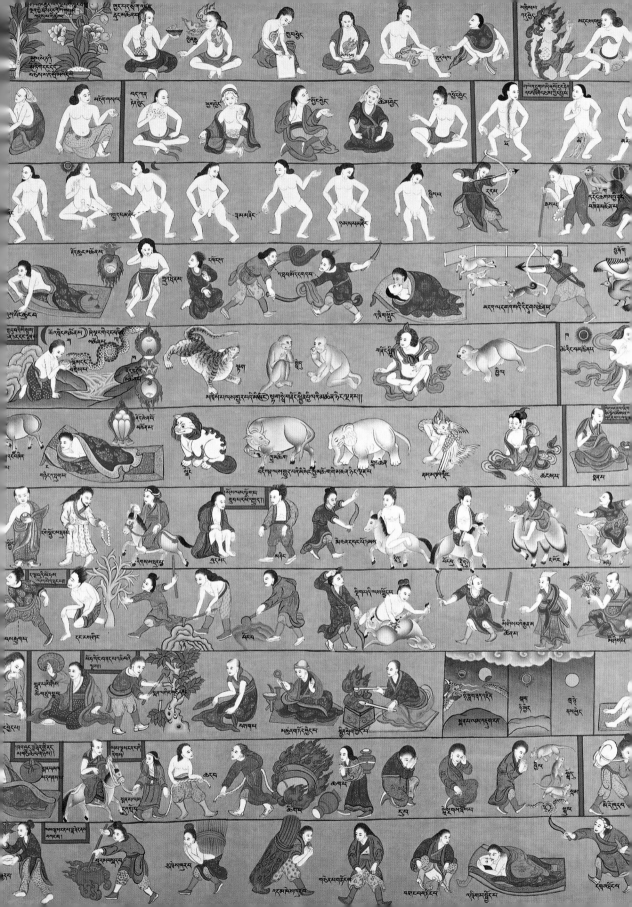

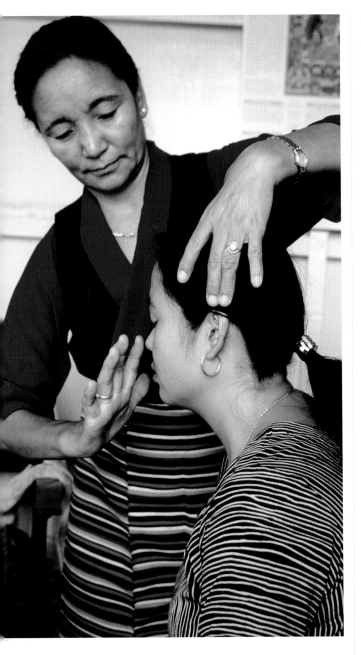

Consultation is required to establish the exact combination of energies that make up your constitutional type.

out in summer and subside in autumn. *Bekan* diseases begin in winter, break out in spring and subside in summer. *Tripa* diseases begin in summer, break out in autumn and subside in winter. To keep in good health at these different times of year, it is necessary to adjust your diet and behaviour in accordance with the needs of the seasons (see page 96).

The five elements

Everything in the universe is made up of the five elements of earth, water, fire, air and space. Earth provides form; water provides lubrication; fire looks after the proper assimilation of food; air helps the circulation of blood and fluids; and space assists the elements to coexist.

Identifying your constitutional type

Each person's individual metabolism is based both on genetic inheritance and on his or her combination of the three *nyepa* energies. The latter is partly determined before conception by previous karma and partly at conception, depending on the *nyepa* types of the parents. If both parents are *tripa*, for example, then the likelihood is that the baby will be *tripa* too.

To determine your constitutional type, a Tibetan doctor will do a pulse diagnosis and a urine analysis, as well as taking astrological information and a detailed medical history (including that of your parents). However, simple observation of your physical shape and character will enable you to judge which of the three broad energy types is yours (see box). You can then make dietary and lifestyle changes accordingly (see pages 92–99).

In Tibetan medicine, there are a total of seven constitutional types, which may be based around a single *nyepa* energy or be a combination of energies. The best constitution is said to be one that is combined, because then the body and mind are in balance.

a role in memory and concentration. An imbalance of *bekan* may result in ailments that present with oedema and mucus, and it is also associated with diabetes.

Energy and the seasons

Diseases associated with the three energy forces are said to begin in one season, break out in another and subside in a third season. For example, *lung* diseases begin in spring, break

Basic constitutional types

Although you need to consult a doctor of Tibetan medicine to establish exactly how the three energies combine to create your constitutional type, you can get a good indication of which energy predominates from your body shape and other physical characteristics. This will enable you to make some simple dietary changes even if you don't have access to a trained doctor.

Lung types

You are probably thin, with a cold constitution, as well as highly active mentally, talkative and quarrelsome. You tend to suffer from stress and anxiety, insomnia and depression. When your bodily energies are out of balance, your digestion is the first area to be affected, and sleep problems are also likely to ensue.

Tripa types

You are likely to be rounded in body shape and often to feel hungry and thirsty, having a healthy appetite. You sweat easily and may have a strong body odour. You are quick on the uptake and convincing in arguments. Jealousy and anger may well be close to the surface. Your physical weak points are your liver, gallbladder and small intestine. In general you may suffer from hot diseases, which manifest on the skin in particular.

Bekan types

You probably have a strong build (and may be overweight), a cool body and a thick skin. You can endure hunger and thirst and you love your sleep. Your digestion tends to be sluggish, which makes you susceptible to mucus diseases. You may be shy. Of the three nyepa types, you tend to hold onto your wealth the most effectively.

Buddhist concepts of disease

The root of all disease, according to the Buddha, is belief in the self, referred to as marigpa. Buddhist teaching states that as soon as there is belief in this self, there is 'other' and so comes about 'duality', which is experienced as subjectivity, a feeling of separateness and a lack of compassion.

This delusional way of relating to oneself and the world throws the three *nyepa* energies (see page 50) out of balance and thus brings about disease. Fortunately – so Tibetan doctors teach – coming to a Buddhist understanding of the true nature of the universe reverses this process and leads to perfect health.

Who we are

Our sense of our 'self' as a single entity is incorrect, taught the Buddha. We are, in fact, made up of five parts or *skandhas*: form, feeling, perception, thought and consciousness. Self is not solid; we are composed of different components, rather than being solid individuals. Therefore, attending to a delusory solid 'I' – grasping at a self that fundamentally does not exist – is the cause of all suffering and the root of disease. It is thought to give rise to 84,000 *kleshas*, or afflictive emotions. These can be condensed into five types: desire, aversion, ignorance, pride and jealousy. From this delusory mind-set also arise the three mind-poisons – attachment, hatred and ignorance – that cause the three *nyepa* energies to fall out of balance. When *lung*, *tripa* or *bekan* becomes excessive by being aggravated by its corresponding mind-poison (attachment affects *lung*, anger affects *tripa* and ignorance affects *bekan*), the result is disease.

Stress and disease

Tibetan medicine regards the predominant cause of health complaints to be an imbalance of *lung*. This tends to be caused by attachment or craving.

Attachment to selfish desire and not wanting to accept that the very nature of the universe is change and impermanence leads, over time, to grief, which Tibetan doctors consider to be a much-ignored symptom in the West that causes stress and suffering. This way of thinking about health has implications for the many diseases of the Western world that are stress-related – a reported eight out of ten of the most commonly prescribed medications in the United States are used to manage stress disorders, from depression and anxiety to high blood pressure and digestive problems. Tibetan doctors say that the Western model of living, which defines success by material possessions or physiological states such as extreme thinness, gives rise to *lung* disorders. Studies suggest that such cravings do not bring contentment. Though we in the West may be richer in possessions than we were 50 years ago, research shows that we do not consider ourselves any happier.

Tibetan medicine may be so effective because it accepts as a fundamental part of its structure that all diseases are *lung*-derived and therefore psychosomatic in nature. For Tibetan doctors, treatment therefore begins with the introduction and explanation to the patient of *shunyata*, or emptiness-awareness. *Shunyata*, they profess, is the true nature of reality and the supreme medicine, because it eradicates the root cause of the three mind-poisons – grasping at a self that fundamentally does not exist. Uprooting this tendency pacifies all forms of disease. Only by transforming a patient from fixation on the self-grasping *marigpa* to a world view of openness or selflessness (*rigpa*) can disease be fundamentally and permanently conquered.

The four mind benders

The 'four mind benders' (which come from a set of Tibetan Buddhist sayings known as the Lojong Preliminaries) are used to generate a search for

In Buddhist thought, physical health is gained by reaching an understanding of the true illusory nature of the world.

complete freedom, which can only be obtained by genuine study of the *Dharma*. When you know the reality and truth of these statements, a genuine attitude of renunciation arises in your mind towards practice and you see the true reality devoid of self:

'*Life is precious*
Death comes without warning
Karma cannot be escaped
Egocentricity is the root of all suffering.'

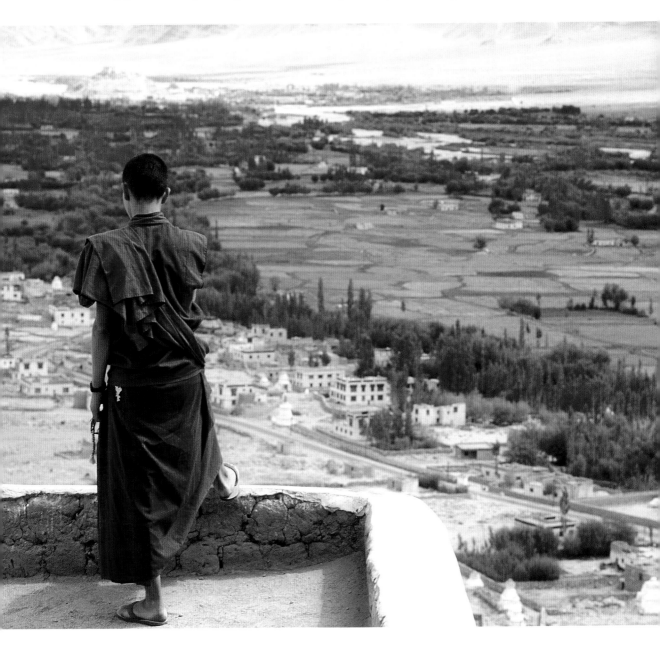

Chakras: psychic energy wheels

Chakra is the Sanskrit word meaning 'wheel'. Known as khor-lo *in Tibetan, the term refers to the energy centres in the body, which have been used for centuries by Tantric yogis to achieve enlightenment. Modern science has established that these energy centres correspond closely to nerve ganglia in the body, and each one is located near a glandular system that produces hormones determining the state of metabolism, sleep, reproduction, immunity and mental health. Nobel Prize-winning doctor Alexis Carrel calls the glandular system the 'wheel of life' that sustains all cellular functions in the human body.*

How they work

These powerful centres of energy are created where the *roma* and *rkyan ma* side-channels carrying *tsog-lung* vital force intersect around the central *uma* channel (see page 48). The chakras act as pumps or valves that regulate the flow of energy throughout the body.

Tibetan Buddhism focuses on five chakras, rather than the seven of the Hindu tradition. Tibetan medicine uses six – the extra one being the wisdom-eye chakra at the brow. This chakra is also known as the third-eye chakra.

Tantric yogis perform secret practices that cause the mystic fire known as *tummo*, which is produced at the navel chakra, to rise up the central channel, opening the chakras as it passes up through them until it reaches the uppermost chakra at the crown of the head. Tantric adepts believe that when the mystic fire *tummo* reaches the white drop that inhabits this chakra, bliss results and enlightenment is achieved. Another name for this chakra is the Wheel of Bliss. When fully opened, the chakras serve as internal mandalas of Five Dhayani Buddhas (see page 58). It is said that when Padmasambhava went to find a yogini, he first met her student and attendant who cut open her chest to reveal the Buddha fields within.

Extremely accomplished chakra practices, such as the Six Yogas of Naropa (see page 144), permit adults to enter the inner worlds that children access so effortlessly. Some thinkers believe that this is because such practices stimulate the thymus and pineal glands, which atrophy after childhood, leading to increased self-consciousness.

'The chakras act as pumps or valves that regulate the flow of energy throughout the body'

The chakra system

Each chakra is associated with a sacred syllable: *Om* (crown chakra); *Ah* (throat chakra); *Hung* (heart chakra); *Hrih* (navel chakra); *Ma* (sexual chakra). The syllable of the wisdom-eye chakra is secret.

Crown chakra

The highest of the body's chakras is situated at the crown of the head and activating it through *tummo* clears the body of negative karma. This chakra is white in colour. It is located at the pituitary gland, which is sometimes called the master gland because it has influence over all the other hormone-producing glands in the body.

Wisdom-eye chakra

This is located on the forehead, from where it controls the eyes, nerves, head and brain in the physical body and also generates telepathy, clairvoyance and precognition. The pineal gland is situated at this centre, producing melatonin, which regulates the sleep cycle. Another function of this gland is release of dimethyltryptamine (DMT), known as the 'spirit molecule'. DMT is always present in the body, but at birth, death and perhaps enlightenment it is released. It is believed to be connected with mystical experiences.

Throat chakra

Situated at the throat, this chakra is the seat of the thyroid gland in the physical body, which produces thyroxine, a hormone that regulates metabolism. This chakra is red in colour. Its role concerns speech and self-expression and it is involved in the transmutation of desire.

Heart chakra

Located at the thymus gland, this chakra is linked in the physical body to the thymus gland, which controls the immune system. Its colour is blue. This is considered to be the seat of the mind and is concerned with the transmutation of anger. The energies from this centre affect the heart, lungs, upper chest, back and bronchial tubes.

Navel chakra

Found just below the bellybutton, this chakra is linked to the digestive system, including the pancreas, liver and stomach. It is yellow in colour. When this centre is activated by Tantric adepts through sacred practices, it produces the mystic heat known as *tummo*, which is said to blow away the belief in the self and thus bring about enlightenment.

Sexual chakra

Based at the hip and genital region, this chakra is the seat of the vital energy, *lung*. In the Tibetan tradition it is visualized as green. The negative mental state, or 'mind-poison', of desire (or attachment to objects and emotions) is based in the sexual chakra.

Revealing our divine nature

Both religious and medical Tantric practices have the same goal: purifying the subtle body of blockages and knots of negative energy that keep us from health and enlightenment. This is why there is no separation between religion and medicine in the Tibetan culture.

Tantric adepts may appear as ordinary beings, but internally they have realized the five Buddha fields of the chakras and have become emanations of particular deities.

At the five chakras lie the five 'mind-poisons' (three main ones, plus two minor ones) that Tibetan medicine believes lead directly to illness: pride, aversion, anger, greed and jealousy. By doing guru yoga, mantras and *tummo* inner-heat yoga (see page 144), the poisons are transmuted into the five wisdoms, which are described as follows: mirror-like, equanimity, *dharmadatu* (the 'ground of Buddhahood'), discerning and all accomplishing. The poisons also become transformed into the Five Dhyani Buddhas: Vairochana, Aksobhya, Ratnasambhava, Amitabha and Amogasiddhi.

This illustration represents the way absolute mind-essence spreads through the body as tigle *essences.*

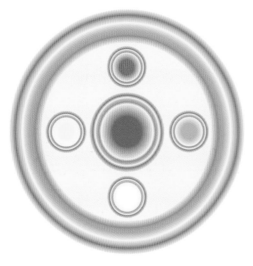

Performing the medicine practice

Forty-two peaceful deities reside in the heart centre and 58 wrathful deities in the head centre. To try the practice of the Medicine Buddha, visualize the Medicine Buddha at your crown chakra and the Medicine Mountains at the other four chakras as follows: Malaya at the throat chakra, maintaining the vital organs; Ponadan, which cures every disease, at the heart chakra; Begche, which neutralizes heat, at the navel chakra; and Gangchen, which also neutralizes heat, at the genital chakra. In this way you gradually make your body into a microcosm of the Medicine Buddha's paradise (see page 106).

The heart drop of life

The absolute mind-essence or *bodhicitta* drop is located at the heart centre, but it spreads through the body in *tigle* essences that are made up of the body's vital essences, such as semen. These essences are drawn through the *rtsa* energy channels into the base of the central *uma* channel, where, at the navel chakra, they are purified and transmuted by mystic fire, or *tummo*, from blocking negative mind-poisons into positive, liberating wisdoms. As the *tigle* essences melt, they cause an upward flow of heat that opens up the chakras, revealing mandalas, or symbolic diagrams, of the Five Dhyani Buddhas. When the flow reaches the crown chakra at the

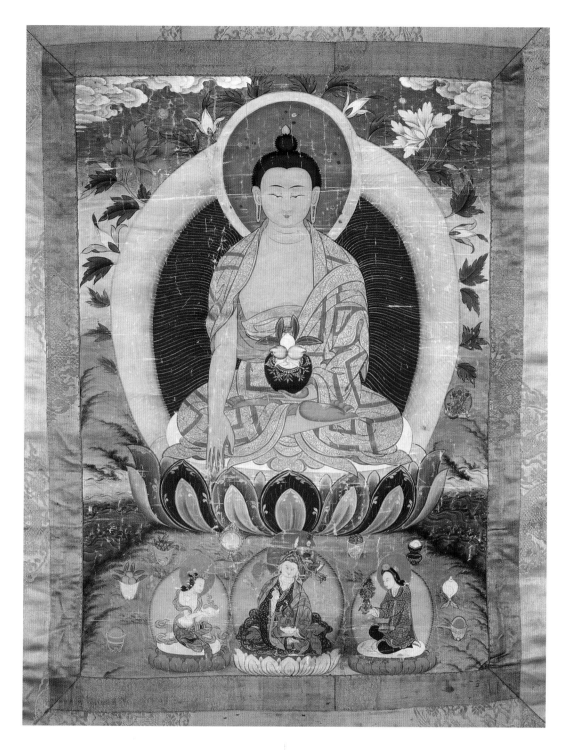

head, bliss is experienced and all notion of a separate self – *marigpa* – melts away, dissolving disease and suffering.

The heart *tigle* or *mdang-chhog*, from which all *tigle* essences derive, is made up of five lights, said to be your innate Buddha nature. This does

During the healing medicine meditation practice, the Medicine Buddha is visualized at the crown chakra.

not have to be developed through practice, but rather is revealed, since your Buddha nature cannot be cultivated, but is always there.

The role of the environment

All the great Eastern medical texts describe the key role of an individual's environment in the promotion of health and wellbeing. The Medicine Buddha's mandala sits at the centre of Tibetan medicine as a metaphor of the healing role of a protected and pure environment, free of pollutants. When nature is in harmony, all its produce is medicine and our planet becomes a healing biosphere. And so, to ensure the health of humanity, we must protect the wellbeing of the planet.

A healing paradise

Tibetan medicine teaches that if the environment is polluted, the five elements that make up the universe and ourselves become imbalanced, giving rise to physical, mental and emotional ill health. Commentators note how the recent rise in the incidence of diseases such as cancer and depression mirrors the growth of environmental destruction and increased pollution brought about by widespread industrialization.

For many centuries, Tibet was an unpolluted environment, and generations of doctors picked plants on its plateaux to create their herbal formulas. Many Tibetan doctors report that it is now difficult to find medicinal plants that are unpolluted by the industrial smoke-stacks to the west of Tibet, while other healing herbs are over-farmed to supply the demands of mainland China. Indeed, every day across the globe, hundreds of species of healing plants are lost for ever through the destruction of rainforests and other natural habitats – and with them the indigenous people who have knowledge of their medicinal uses. Animals are also being driven to extinction by humankind's treatment of the environment, whether by oil spills or the invisible pollution of habitats by persistent use of chemicals, which are shown to 'feminize' male animals by mimicking the effects of oestrogen.

We urgently need to explore means of conserving the world's resources, such as the plants that may hold the key to the medicine of future generations. One important way in which you can help preserve the environment (as well as benefit your own health) is to choose organic food. If this choice is repeated by many people on a daily basis, the small actions of individuals will together prevent the use of many tons of pesticides. Tibetan medicine urges us to conserve natural habitats and show compassion for all sentient beings.

Water and good health

The *Gyud Zhi* lists seven types of water – rain, melted snow, river, spring, well, sea and forest water – but says the most important for health is 'living water' from an unpolluted source exposed to the elements of nature. Japanese studies of water crystals have demonstrated that water sourced from mountain streams or sacred places has a greater ability to form water crystals, while the worst results come from tap water and water that is polluted. Groundwater polluted with agricultural and industrial chemicals, and tap water adulterated with fluoride or chlorine, are

Tibetan medicine teaches the importance of protecting our environment, in particular natural sources of water.

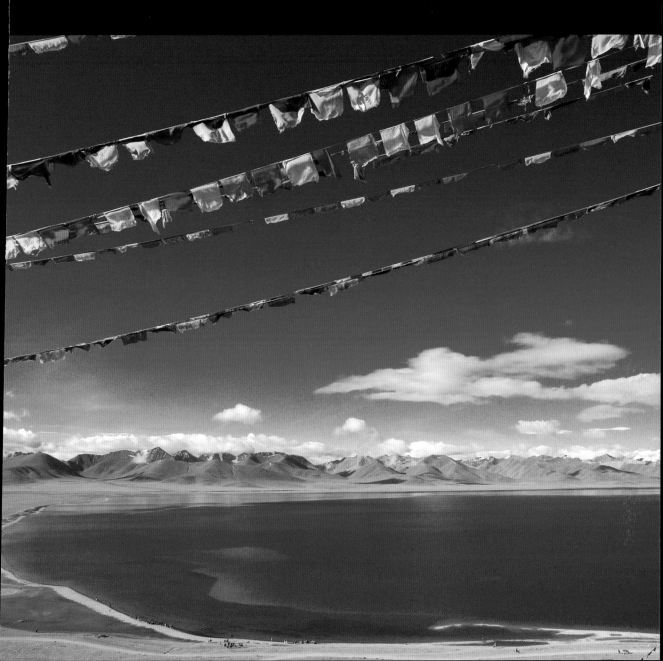

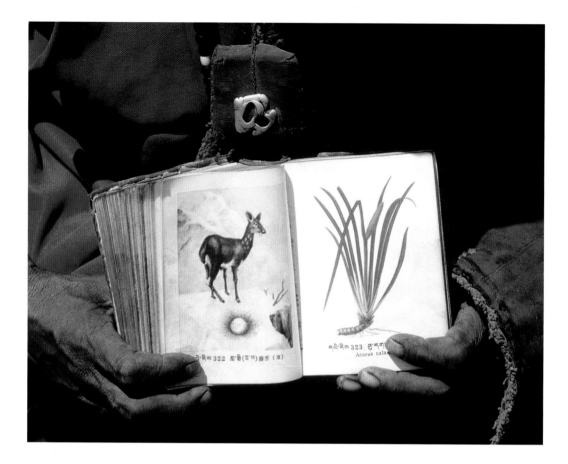

all thought by Tibetan doctors to pollute the microcosm of the body as they do the macrocosm of the earth.

Polluted land and air

Heavy metals released by industrial processes, such as mercury, lead and cadmium, accumulate in the environment and pass into our bodies through repeated exposure over time to car-exhaust emissions, sources in the home such as old paint, and foods such as fish. They contribute to a number of well-defined diseases, including birth defects and brain and behavioural disorders. Doctors of Tibetan medicine may recommend a form of chelation therapy that removes such heavy metals from the body (see page 113).

Naga diseases

Doctors of Tibetan medicine also monitor the effects of environmental pollution on an invisible world. *Nagas*, earth spirits and guardians of

Tibetan doctors draw on the natural world for remedies that for centuries have been used effectively to treat human ills.

place, have long been thought to protect spiritual practitioners. A *naga* sheltered the Buddha as he meditated, for example, protecting him from the elements with his hood. Although unseen by the physical eye, these potent elemental forces are certainly felt by those who believe in them.

In Tibetan medicine 360 diseases are said to be caused by *nagas*, which are snake-like in nature and give rise to diseases linked to an imbalance of *bekan* energy. When their habitats are polluted, these spirits are said to cause diseases including AIDS and cancer, and to cause environmental disasters such as earthquakes and tidal waves. When illness comes after a period of perfect health, a patient might be asked if he or she has disturbed the habitat of a *naga*. The cutting down of a tree or removal of stones is reputed to be enough to anger them into provoking disease.

If the damage can be repaired, the disease sometimes curiously disappears. When they and their environment are respected, these spirits may bestow wealth, treasures and spiritual gifts and Tibetans sometimes attribute good fortune to blessings from the *nagas* (see page 111 for how to make an offering to appease the *nagas*).

Treasure vases

Padmasambhava gave special secret instructions for the creation of treasure vases (*terbum*) to help the practitioners of *Dharma*. There are two types of treasure vases: wealth vases and earth vases.

Wealth vases are created with many precious things, such as crystals, jewels, mandala pictures of wealth deities, mantras and special pills. Having such a vase in the home is said to bring good fortune, prosperity (both material and spiritual) and good relationships with people.

Earth vases, when blessed and activated, can affect the environment for 24 km (15 miles) around, and are normally buried in the ground to restore the earth's life force. They are prepared with conch shells, turquoises, crystals, cowrie shells and iron pyrite, and they impart life essence to gods, humans, *nagas*, *dakinis* (female deities) and local protectors, and to the *Dharma* practitioners in the area.

Earth vases are also said to restore the five elements of the environment, from which all things are composed, and to impart healing to *nagas* for the pain and suffering caused by pollution. Earth vases generate good health, long life, plentiful harvests, environmental protection and peace.

Authentic treasure vases are sealed and consecrated in a seven-day ceremony with prayers by many monks and high lamas. The vases must not be touched directly by hand, and should be placed in a display case on a shrine in the home. The seal must never be broken. In the past, vases – particularly earth vases – were made by great masters who had the power to stop war, famine and disease. Today, treasure vases can be purchased from Tsem Tulku

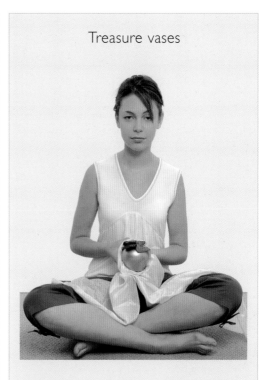

Treasure vases

A treasure vase will bring good fortune to your home and may also be used as a focus of meditation. Do not touch it directly with your fingers but instead cover your hand with a cloth, such as a silk scarf, before lifting it.

monastery in Malaysia, while earth vases can be bought from the Ewam Choden Tibetan Buddhist Center in California.

The Tibetan solution

Buddhists point out that the world's current environmental crisis vividly depicts how the actions of humankind – from industrial revolution to war – cannot escape the karmic principles of cause and effect. The Dalai Lama's vision for the future of Tibet could be a blueprint for environmental protection and the sustainability of the world. In 1987 he proposed that Tibet become a peace park for the world: a sanctuary of human rights and non-violence that would help redress global environmental imbalance. May this wish come to fruition.

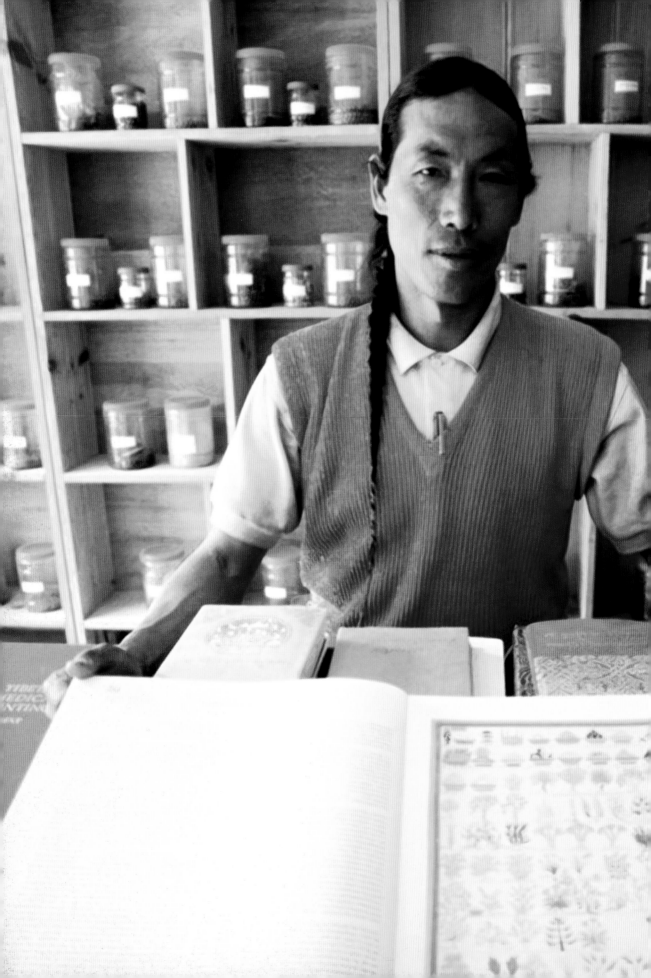

Tools of the Tibetan doctor

Doctors of Tibetan medicine have been carrying out their complex array of diagnostic tests on the roof of the world for centuries. Today, Western doctors are eager to understand how such relatively simple – and inexpensive – tests can give such profound diagnoses. Researchers are providing medical science with modern forms of the ancient Tibetan methods of pulse and urine analysis in a bid to replicate the results in Western settings and reduce the side-effects of conventional medication. Other diagnostic tools, such as divination, are less tangible to Western ways of thinking. To know Tibetan medicine is to understand it as a profound system of enlightenment.

Pulse diagnosis

One of the most fascinating and skilful diagnostic methods used in Tibetan medicine is pulse diagnosis. The practice of pulse diagnosis functions like a three-way telephone conversation between the doctor, the organs and the body's energetic constitution. Simply feeling a pulse is routine in Western medicine, but in Tibetan medicine doctors listen to the pulse. To learn the basics of pulse diagnosis takes one year, while to master the art proficiently requires a decade at the very least.

Western evaluation

In the 1970s the American surgeon Dr Richard Selzer, who practised at Yale Medical School until he retired in 1986, spent time observing Dr Yeshi Dhonden (see page 34) as he carried out pulse diagnosis. Dr Selzer described this present-day Medicine Buddha as a living MRI scanner. Dr Dhonden proved that he was repeatedly able to diagnose disease using simply the highly attuned tips of his fingers. In some cases he outperformed contemporary scientific equipment and medical tests, for example by stating to which organ a tumour had started to spread. In *Mortal Lessons*, Dr Selzer described what he had seen: 'He felt her pulse for a long, long time. He parted from us, really. Then he emerged to give, in this metaphoric way, the exact diagnosis. I was completely floored.'

The diagnostic method

According to Tantric anatomy, there are three main channels in the body transporting vital force: *rkyan ma*, *roma* and *uma* (see page 48). *Rkyan ma*, where *bekan* energy predominates, is under the influence of the moon. *Roma*, where *tripa* energy predominates, is under the influence of the sun. *Uma*, which is associated with *lung* energy, is neutral. Therefore, the best time for pulse diagnosis is said to be early in the morning when the two energies influenced by the cold of night and the warmth of day – *bekan* and *tripa* – are at an equivalent level.

The doctor starts to read a male patient's heart pulse on the patient's left arm, feeling the wrist with the fingers of the right hand. If the patient is a woman, the doctor starts to read the heart pulse using his or her left hand on the patient's right arm. This is because the tip of the female heart is situated towards the right of the body and that of the male towards the left. And so, in Tibetan medicine, the right side of the body represents emptiness, or *shunyata*, the feminine principle, while the left side of the body represents skilful means, relating to *upaya*, the masculine principle. The other pulses to which the doctor listens are in the same position for both male and female patients (see page 68). Six pulses are taken in total, three on each arm.

The doctor then tries to determine an overall picture of the patient's health from the pulse information he or she has gathered. Listening to the pulse illustrates what is happening in the patient's five internal organs and six cavities in the upper and lower parts of the body (the stomach, small intestine, large intestine,

By taking pulses on the left and right wrists, a doctor can build up a complex picture of the patient's internal organs.

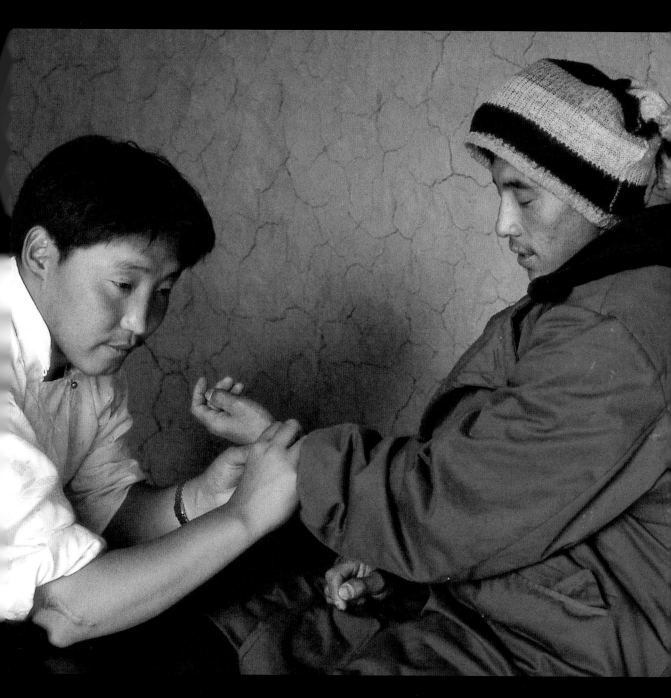

'I know that I, one who has taken
thousands of pulses, have never
felt a single one'

From *Mortal Lessons*, Richard Selzer

PULSE DIAGNOSIS   67

What the pulses reveal

In a man, the heart pulse is read on the left wrist and the lung pulse
on the right wrist; in a woman these positions are reversed. The other
pulses are in the same position for men and women.

Taking the pulse on the left wrist

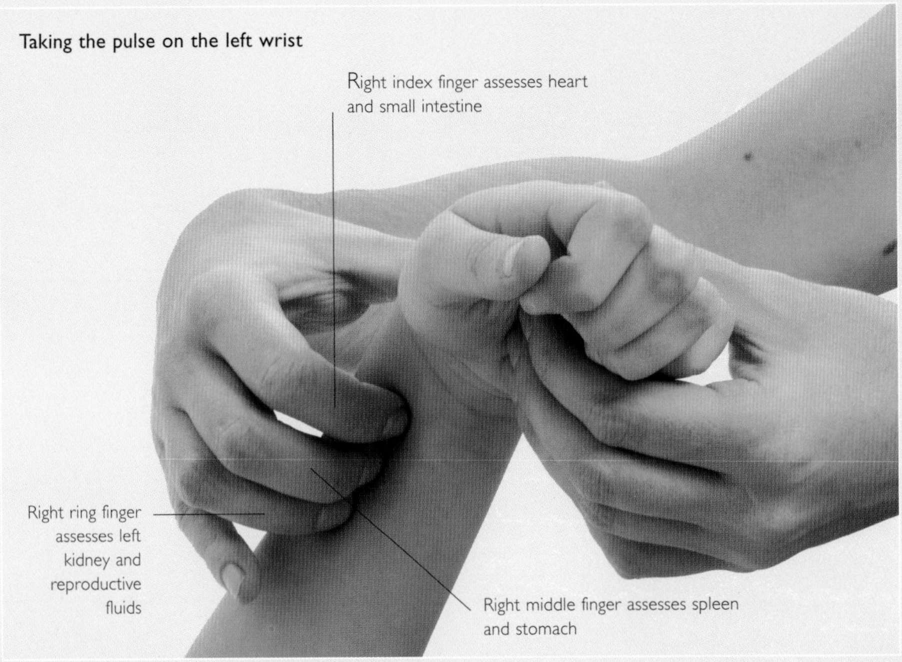

Right index finger assesses heart
and small intestine

Right ring finger
assesses left
kidney and
reproductive
fluids

Right middle finger assesses spleen
and stomach

Taking the pulse on the right wrist

Left index finger assesses lungs and
large intestine

Left middle finger assesses
liver and gallbladder

Left ring finger assesses right
kidney and bladder

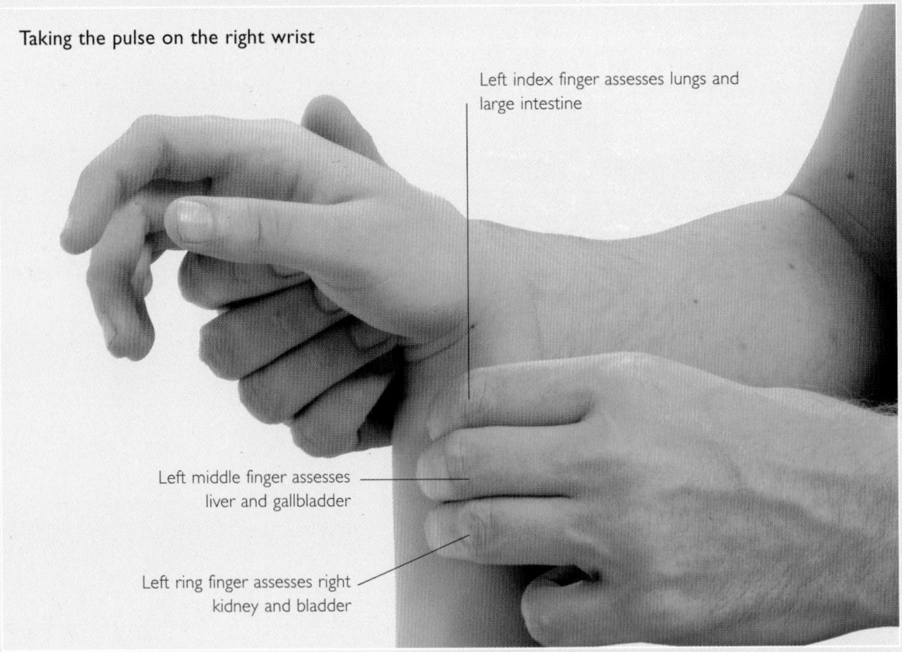

gallbladder, urinary bladder and reproductive organs, including the breasts), in the three *nyepa* energies (*lung*, *bekan* and *tripa*) and in the five elements within the body (earth, air, water, fire and space).

The qualities of the pulse

The fourth *tantras* of the *Gyud Zhi* states that there are three constitutional pulses: male, female and neutral (known as the *bodhisattva* pulse), and each is defined by specific qualities, which are secret and known only to doctors trained in Tibetan medicine. These tell doctors whether the three life energies are in balance, whether the patient's disease is 'hot' or 'cold' and whether someone is suffering from spirit possession. A healthy person has five heart beats that repeat with regularity over one minute. A pulse rate over five beats per minute indicates that the patient has a 'hot' disease; a pulse rate with fewer than five beats a minute indicates a 'cold' disease. Beats of ten per minute – or even one single beat – indicate a serious condition. Traditionally, an irregular beat is seen as a sign of demonic possession.

The three *nyepa* pulses

As there are three different energies in the subtle body – *lung*, *tripa* and *bekan* – so there are three energetic pulses. The *lung* pulse has a floating or drifting quality and is easily felt. There is an unpredictability about a *lung* pulse – if the doctor exerts pressure on the blood vessel, the pulse disappears, like a ball being pushed under water; when the pressure is released, the pulse returns. A *tripa* pulse is easily recognized since it bangs against the artery wall, indicating pressure and perhaps tension. A *bekan* pulse has a sunken feeling and a thickness like honey or glue; being weak, it has fewer than five pulse beats per minute. Each type of pulse indicates that the person in question belongs to that constitution and should live and eat accordingly.

The Seven Astonishing Pulses

Certain doctors of Tibetan medicine who have mastered the art of pulse diagnosis evolve to such a level of consciousness, training and karma that they are blessed with the clairvoyant healing ability of the Seven Astonishing Pulses: an ability to determine future events in the life of a patient. These predictions concern a patient's family, guests, enemies, friends and also evil spirits. Such doctors may be able to diagnose a family member unable to attend the surgery.

Pulse diagnosis in modern medicine

In 1960 scientists from the Soviet Union began a long-term study of Tibetan medicine, with a particular focus on the mechanics of pulse diagnosis. This research has led to the development of an automated pulse-reading machine based on the principles of Tibetan medicine. Though this system is less impressive than a healing master, it may prove important in helping Western medical practitioners to come to an understanding of *tsog-lung* vital force and its relevance in the treatment of disease.

'As there are different energies in the body, so there are three energetic pulses'

Urine diagnosis

In a patient's urine a Tibetan doctor sees all the body's metabolic processes reflected. By noting the colour, texture and scent of the urine, the doctor can spot any imbalance in the three energies of lung, bekan *and* tripa, *which indicates disease or disorder within the body. Doctors separate the urine and see which herbs and medicines dissolve or change the nature of the urine. By this process of screening, they determine the best medicine to prescribe to their patients.*

In his book, *Tibetan Medicine*, the Ven. Rechung Rinpoche draws on the *Gyud Zhi* to explain the theory of urine analysis:

'Food is broken down by the bekan *energy, and then digested by the* tripa *energy in the body and the* lung *energy absorbs the nutrients. The digested food goes into the intestines where the sediment goes into the bladder and the liquid portion goes to the stomach where it is transported to the liver and transformed into blood.'*

The diagnostic method

A doctor of Tibetan medicine assesses urine that has been passed at dawn or shortly after, since its colour will then not be affected by waste material from the digestive process. Traditionally, the doctor uses a bamboo whisk to stir the urine. In the medical texts, the urine of a healthy person is described as being like the colour of golden straw, smelling like cream and having average-sized bubbles. Excess of one of the *nyepa* energies is revealed in changes to the colour, smell or texture of the urine (see box). Such changes are used as indicators for diagnosis and treatment.

Mewa urine analysis

In *mewa* urine analysis, the physician examines the urine sample from above, imagining a grid that resembles the nine squares on a turtle's

---

What urine reveals

Lung urine

This has no smell and hardly any steam and, when beaten, large bubbles appear. An excessive *lung* imbalance is indicated by a pale blue colour.

Tripa urine

This is strong-smelling and dark yellow to orange. When stirred, small bubbles form and quickly burst. If a specimen of strong *tripa* urine is left to stand, albumin is found floating as clots. This is *guja*, which looks like a piece of cotton. The level at which it floats in the urine – bottom, middle or top – indicates the site of imbalance in the body.

Bekan urine

Where *bekan* predominates, urine is greyish, foamy and contains small, steady bluish bubbles. A rainbow colouring indicates poisoning.

Sediment in the urine

Sediment indicates *lung* disorders if it can be picked up; heart disease if it floats; and kidney disorder if it settles on the bottom. Scum on the surface of the urine indicates a tumour.

underbelly. This is the same grid used for divination in Tibetan astrology (see page 76). Each of the nine boxes represents an astrological influence on the patient, which are categorized as gods, humans, demons, cremation area, house, natural environment, ancestors, patient's life spirit and offspring. Whichever influence is shown in a section of the projected grid may need to be 'antidoted' through religious practice. This type of diagnostic method is one of the most difficult practices of Tibetan medicine to learn and understand.

Urine diagnosis in modern medicine

Tibetan medicine uses the information contained in a patient's urine to describe his or her state of health, but until recently this source of data has been largely ignored by Western medicine. However, Western doctors do already test urine for eight factors – urobilinogen, protein, pH levels, blood, glucose, ketones, bilirubin and specific gravity – and certain substances that the test detects, such as blood, are considered to be potential signs of disease.

Western medicine has also recently begun to use the results of urine analysis as a means of personalizing drug treatment. Through examination of a patient's urine, the levels of his or her tolerance to certain drugs can be established, because drug-tolerance levels are genetically based and influenced by internal biochemical factors, such as gut bacteria.

Professor Jeremy Nicholson and his colleagues at Imperial College London have devised a urine test that analyses excreted metabolites (small molecules produced naturally by the body). Their research has shown that the individual metabolite make-up of urine reflects a patient's genetic and biochemical profile. This is proof in Western scientific terms of something that Tibetan medicine has known for centuries.

Researchers using urine metabolite profiling to prevent drug toxicity have found that the method outperforms older practices in new drug tests. It would be a small step from here to use this

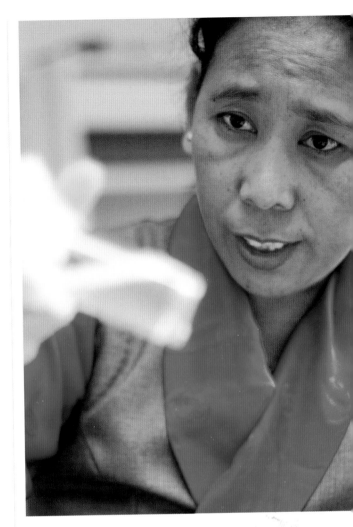

The colour, texture and scent of urine reflect how well the three energies are balanced and the patient's state of health.

knowledge to develop a test to determine a patient's constitution according to the principles of Tibetan medicine.

Tibetan medicine teaches that metabolite excretions in urine can reveal the earliest stages of disease. Urine tests provide more accurate information than blood tests, which don't register disease until it has reached chronic levels. Researchers in Italy, for example, have found that a urine test for the enzyme telomerase (which is found in high levels in cancer cells) can detect bladder cancer to 90 per cent accuracy. This non-invasive technique has much to offer in the treatment of bladder cancer.

Tongue diagnosis

The tongue has been used as a tool of medical diagnosis since the Shang Dynasty in China in 1,000 BCE. For many trained physicians and healers, the tongue is the window into the body and its functions — and, even when untrained, we can get a revealing insight into our current state of health by checking our tongue each morning. If it does not look healthy, you might like to visit a qualified Tibetan doctor to find out why.

What the tongue reveals

Until late into the 19th century, examining the tongue was an orthodox diagnostic tool for Western doctors, who believed that sections of the tongue were connected to organs in the body and so revealed their condition. Tibetan medicine also analyses the tongue in terms of its zones and related parts of the body. It also examines the coating of the tongue, which comes about as a result of the digestive process and so can be used by a trained physician to assess the condition of the patient's digestion. In a patient where *lung* energy predominates, the tongue is red and dry with bumps on the sides. A *tripa* tongue is noted for its yellow coating. A *bekan* tongue is pale with a sticky white coating.

The diagnostic method

Tongue analysis is not a primary diagnostic tool in Tibetan medicine, but is used largely to confirm what the doctor has determined from pulse and urine diagnosis. Tibetan medicine regards the tongue as a map of the internal body. When a doctor examines a patient's tongue, he or she looks primarily for signs that reveal the health of the three vital forces — *lung, tripa* and *bekan* — and then for indicators of the digestive system and the efficiency of mineral absorption from food. Doctors may also note signs of stress displayed on the tongue.

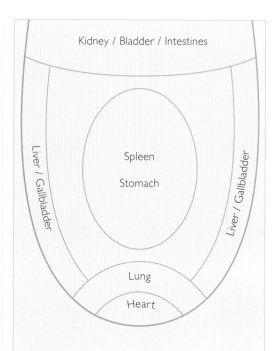

Zones of the tongue

Tibetan medicine treats the tongue as a map of the body, with zones reflecting the health of specific organs. The tip of the tongue is linked to the heart and lungs, for example, while its sides both reflect the liver and gallbladder, its central zone the spleen and stomach and its back area the kidneys, bladder and intestines.

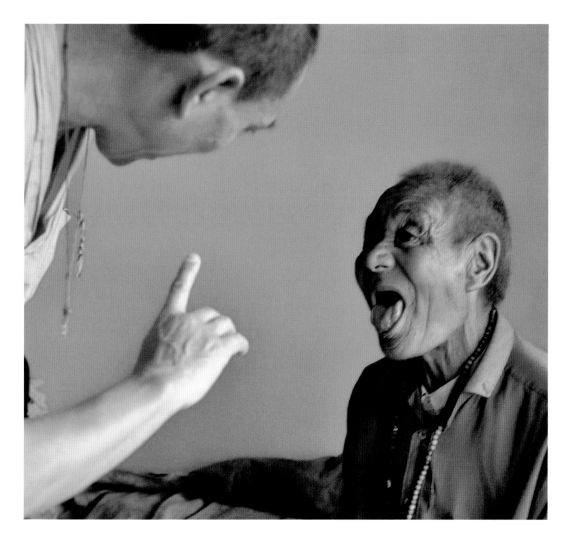

Tongue diagnosis in modern medicine

In 1987, after a study that recorded the state of the tongues of 12,000 patients, scientists reported in the *Chinese Journal of Oncology* that the colour and coating of the tongues of cancer patients were found to be significantly different from those of healthy individuals. A group of researchers at the University of Pittsburgh is

The appearance of the tongue illustrates the patient's overall wellbeing as well as the condition of different organs.

now experimenting with using tongue diagnosis as a method of early diagnosis in the detection of colon cancer. The Pittsburgh team are using computerized images of patients' tongues in order to try to determine early cancer profiles.

'Tongue diagnosis is used largely to confirm the results of pulse and urine diagnosis'

Astrological diagnosis

Tibetan astrological texts used to diagnose and treat disease date from as early as the 7th century CE. The system developed through the fusing of the Kalachakra Tantra (the Tantric calendar) with thinking from other systems, including Chinese and Hindu astrology. In Tibet, astrologers have been valued as highly as Tibetan doctors and are traditionally consulted about marriage, birth and death dates and auspicious times for projects such as starting a business, as well as about sickness. They are even called on to develop weather forecasts and help to find reincarnate lamas.

The wheels of time

Tibetan astrology incorporates the most effective components of the *Kalachakra Tantra*, which was devised to enable practitioners of Tantric Buddhism to ensure that their practice was in harmony with the cosmos. The *Kalachakra Tantra* is a calendar formed from the three wheels of time: outer, inner and secret time. The outer wheel refers to the macrocosm: the planets of our solar system and the cosmos. The inner wheel refers to the wheel of time, psychic channels and their movements and the five elements (earth, air, water, fire and space). The secret wheel represents initiation into the Tantric path of the Kalachakra, whereby the student practises the secret mantra, the generation and completion stages of meditation, the ground to be known, the path to be journeyed and the fruition to be attained – and eventually attains enlightenment. The Kalachakra deity is one of the *yidams* or meditation deities (see page 163) connected with Tibetan medicine and astrology.

Comparison with Western astrology

Whereas Western astrology focuses on a set of personality types, Tibetan astrology assesses a person's entire lifespan. If an individual's astrological chart, which is drawn up through consulting planetary and elemental forces, indicates negative signs, the astrologer can advise on practices and lifestyle changes to prevent negative karma (see page 43) from ripening. Negative karma is considered to be an important source of ill health.

The diagnostic method

A life force known as *la* (see page 11) is said to travel around the body according to the lunar

In their treatment, Tibetan doctors consider the effects of astrological events such as Losar (Buddhist New Year).

'Tibetan astrology focuses not on personality types but on an entire lifespan'

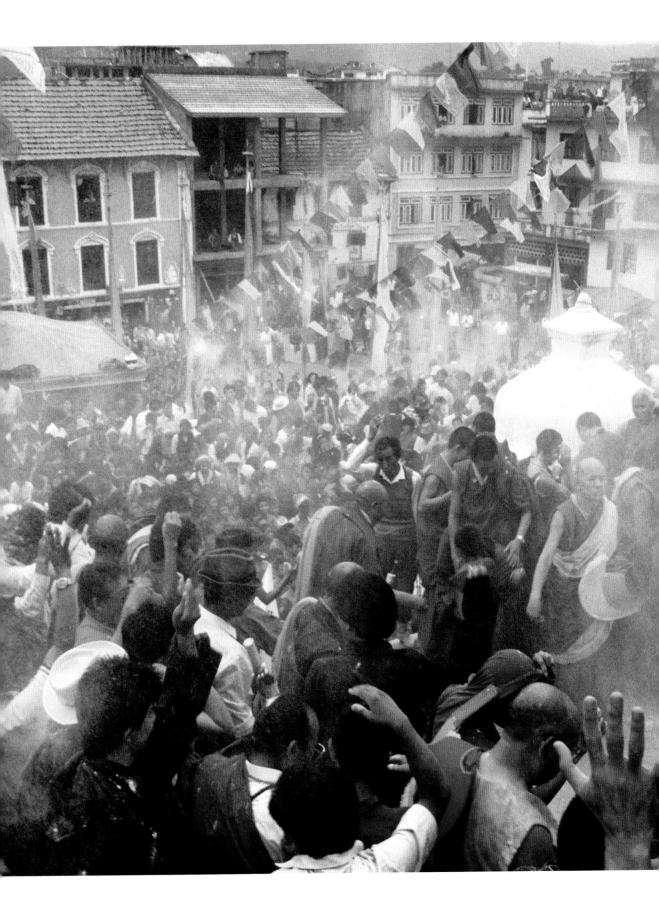

orbit, residing at the crown chakra on the full moon. Astrology enables doctors of Tibetan medicine to establish the exact location of *la* within the body, which they need to know before commencing treatment such as surgery.

During a consultation with a patient, doctors will use a calendar that is derived from the *Kalachakra Tantra* and consists of 360 days divided into seasons. Parts of certain seasons are said to affect the vitality of the organs, and certain days are also specified for their effects on the organs. A Tibetan doctor needs to be aware of these in order to diagnose correctly. The calendar also guides the physician about when to start treatment and the most auspicious time for taking herbal or Precious Jewel Pills (see page 121). Astrological diagnosis also enables a doctor to treat patients who cannot travel for a face-to-face appointment.

The *shipaho* astrological chart

Especially in the treatment of psychiatric disorders (see page 149), doctors of Tibetan medicine may consult an astrological calender to diagnose the force of spirits and their effects on a patient. The *shipaho* astrological chart, a nine-squared grid of magic numbers, is also used by Tibetan doctors, to diagnose *sadakastrologers* or local ground-owner demons.

The *shipaho* chart is found in most Tibetan homes, usually displayed above the main door, such is the high regard in which it is held. It is believed to bring good fortune and health to all who see it. At its centre are the nine squares of magic numbers used in medical diagnosis. The central image of a tortoise represents Manjushri, the deity of wisdom and knowledge, surrounded by flames of wisdom. The 12 animals of the 60-year life cycle (see box, page 78) are also depicted. The Kalachakra mantra, which is used in Tantric practice, is displayed at the top left.

Auspicious practice

When great masters pass away, their passing has an effect on the interdependent energies of the

---

What the calendar reveals

Solar eclipses

At this time, merit gained through practice multiplies significantly. According to Lama Zopa, a high lama who has studied and worked closely with Lama Yeshe since the 1940s, at solar eclipses negative or positive actions are multiplied 100 million times. Therefore, Buddhists try to spend these days praying and chanting.

Lunar eclipses

Merit gained for actions performed during lunar eclipses is said to be multiplied seven million times, so these are also times for prayer and chanting.

Days of Miracles

These first 15 days of the Tibetan calendar are important for religious practice, since all merits at this time are multiplied by 100,000.

Losar or Tibetan New Year

Losar generally occurs around February and is a time of much celebration. During this part of the year, there is also a very important period of religious practice called Chotrul Duchen, which finishes roughly two weeks after Losar. The merit on these days is multiplied and therefore religious practice is observed.

Spirit days

Spirits are more active on certain days of the year, when they may have an adverse effect on the health of individuals.

---

whole planet. They therefore try to choose an auspicious time. For example, Kunsang Denchen Lingpa passed into *parinirvana* on 29 March 2006 at 12.30 am during a solar eclipse. He had been a *terton* who received dream transmissions from Padmasambhava (see page 30).

The lower chakra of this divination thangka *contains a magic square and the animals of Tibetan astrology.*

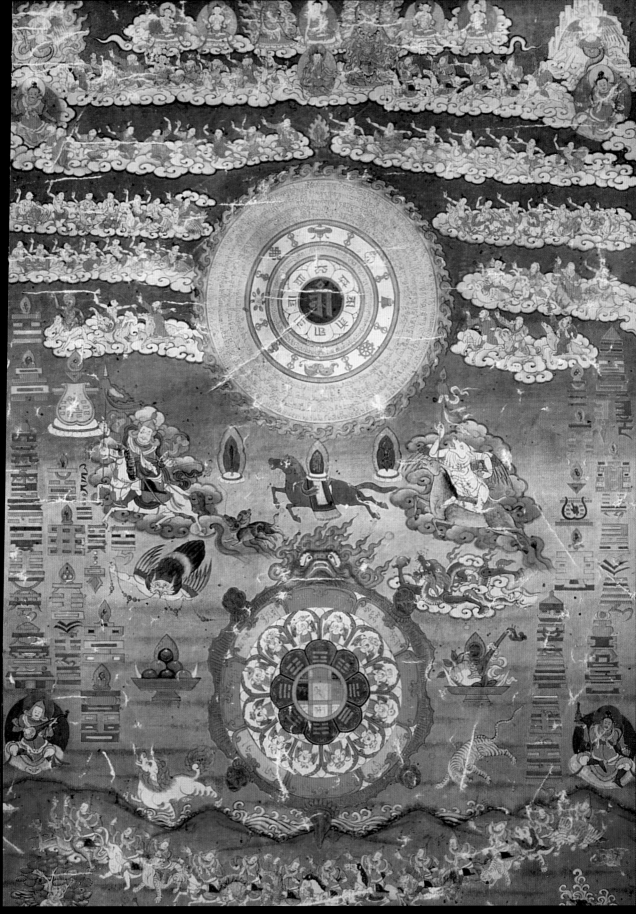

Birth years and associated astrological signs

Dog	1922	1934	1946	1958	1970	1982	1994
Pig	1923	1935	1947	1959	1971	1983	1995
Rat	1924	1936	1948	1960	1972	1984	1996
Ox	1925	1937	1949	1961	1973	1985	1997
Tiger	1926	1938	1950	1962	1974	1986	1998
Hare	1927	1939	1951	1963	1975	1987	1999
Dragon	1928	1940	1952	1964	1976	1988	2000
Snake	1929	1941	1953	1965	1977	1989	2001
Horse	1930	1942	1954	1966	1978	1990	2002
Sheep	1931	1943	1955	1967	1979	1991	2003
Monkey	1932	1944	1956	1968	1980	1992	2004
Bird	1933	1945	1957	1969	1981	1993	2005

Zodiac signs

Tibetan astrology is composed of 12 animal signs. A person's astrological sign is determined by his or her year of birth (see box). Each animal sign represents an element, as well as certain personality traits, such as drive or laziness. Knowing these, the doctor of Tibetan medicine can lead the patient towards health.

Mo divination

The practice of divination has evolved from the incorporation of Tibet's Bon tradition (the spiritual tradition that existed there before the advent of Tantric Buddhism) into the Vajrayana system of Buddhism. This is based on the idea explored in the *Prajnaparamita Sutra* of 'Form is emptiness, emptiness is form', whereby all things are connected. And since all things are interdependent, believers can use divination to attain an unbiased picture of the way things are.

Through a divination reading, someone can determine the successful (or otherwise) outcome of important events such as marriage, business negotiations, house-building or disease, as well as everyday events like the beginning of a journey or the arrival time of a traveller. If the divination reading is not auspicious, spiritual practices such as the liturgy of the Medicine Buddha (see pages 164–169) can be undertaken to stimulate the latent positive forces in the cosmos to bring about a successful outcome. Such practices cannot, however, negate the inevitability that at some point we will all die.

Before doing a divination, a lama or doctor invokes his or her *yidam* or personal deity using a mantra that may, over the course of the lama's lifetime, be recited more than a million times. The lama then asks a question and throws a die with either numbers or letters on its faces and interprets the result using sacred texts. Some healing lamas are so clairvoyant that they need no divination tools. Such is the maturity of their practice and their wisdom that they can see future events and give advice on this basis.

'Divination cannot negate the inevitability that at some point we will all die'

Doing a divination at home

One of the easiest ways to do a divination at home is with a rosary, or prayer beads, as shown below. The answer to your question lies within the number of beads left when you reach the centre of the string, and will be one, two or three beads.

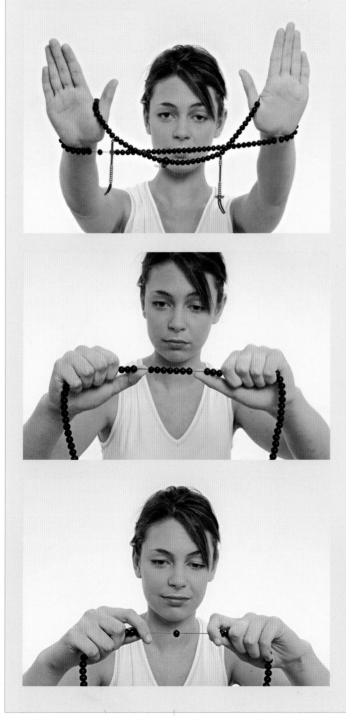

1 Before starting the divination, pray to your deity (see page 163), then ask the question to which you would like an answer. Take the beads in both hands, with the string lying horizontally over your palms, then push your hands forward, hooking the string around your thumbs. Repeat three times, asking your question.

2 Let the rosary fall into your hands. Using the fingers of both hands, move three beads at a time from either side of the centre of the string of beads held between your hands.

3 The number of remaining beads denotes the answer to your question. One bead is a falcon (success), two a raven (defeat) and three a snow lion (a neutral result). Repeat the exercise twice to give three results. Three falcons denotes an excellent outcome.

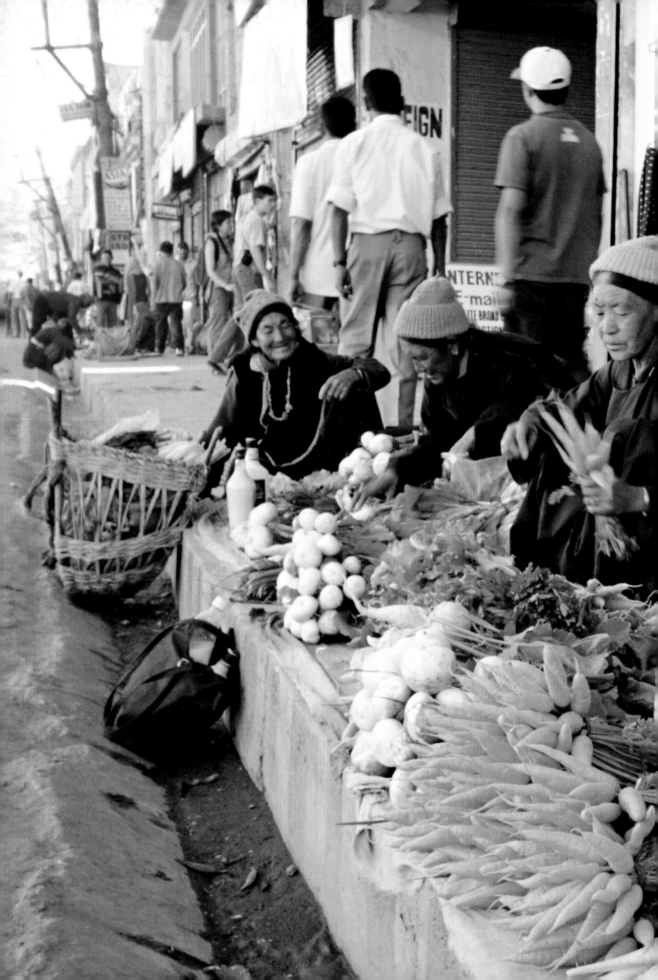

The role of diet in Tibetan medicine

Throughout Asia it is a generally held belief that the best doctor is one who heals patients using food alone. And across the world there is a consensus, both inside and outside the scientific community, that a well-balanced diet ensures good health. Tibetan medicine has always recognized the role of diet in healthcare, believing diet to be one of the four causes of disease and thus a key to its prevention and a powerful treatment. Furthermore, there is an awareness in Tibetan medicine that the goodness of our food reflects the state of our environment: both are at their most health-giving when pure and unpolluted.

Diet in the medical *tantras*

The four medical tantras *of the Gyud Zhi contain very little information about how diet affects health and longevity in a Western sense. The text focuses instead on the ways in which food affects the three vital energies in the body — lung, tripa and bekan (see page 50) — and explains how the five elements in food (earth, air, water, fire and space) give rise to the five elements within the body.*

The digestive process

The medical *tantras* see digestion in terms of an energetic process. *Tripa* is thought to supply heat to the food in the stomach before phlegm breaks it down. The food then separates into two parts: nutrients and waste. The nutrient element moves from the stomach through nine nutrient channels to the liver, where it is turned into the seven bodily constituents that the body needs in order to function properly: nutritional essence (saliva), blood, fat, bone, marrow, flesh and regenerative fluid (which is used for spiritual purposes and ensures vitality). Tibetan medicine teaches that while most food takes a total of six days to be transformed into vital fluid, aphrodisiacs (herbs and foods such as honey, butter, cinnamon and liquorice) take just one hour, which is why they are so highly valued in Tibet.

Qualities and combinations

Food is said to have one of four qualities (it is dry, moist, heavy or light), which have specific effects on the body. Items must also be eaten in the right combination to avoid creating toxicity. For example, eggs are never eaten with fish. Milk and oranges should not be eaten together, nor should milk and meat, as the milk will cause the meat to putrefy in the gut. Melons should be eaten on their own, as they digest rapidly in the body. Sweet fruits, such as banana, should not be eaten with sour fruits, such as pineapple. However, corn and winter squash work well together. Pulses such as lentils need to be eaten with grains to ensure the production of protein.

Digestive heat

Tibetan medicine regards *phet*, or heat in the stomach, as essential to the proper digestion and assimilation of nutrients. Therefore a doctor of Tibetan medicine will advise patients to avoid cold drinks, especially those containing ice, which are thought to smother digestive fire. To restore digestive fire, it is advised to drink ginger tea for about four weeks.

Diet and the constitution

Doctors of Tibetan medicine advise their patients to follow a diet that best suits their individual constitutional type (see page 92). This ensures a balanced mix of the three life forces within the body and thus optimum health. Even if you don't have access to a Tibetan doctor, it is relatively easy to establish whether you are broadly a *lung, tripa* or *bekan* type, based on observation of your physique and character (see page 53). You can then adjust your diet in order to keep the energy forces within you in balance.

Rules of eating

Tibetan medicine requires that you avoid over-eating, as this taxes the body. When eating, you are advised to fill half the stomach with food and another quarter with fluid, reserving one quarter for space to digest.

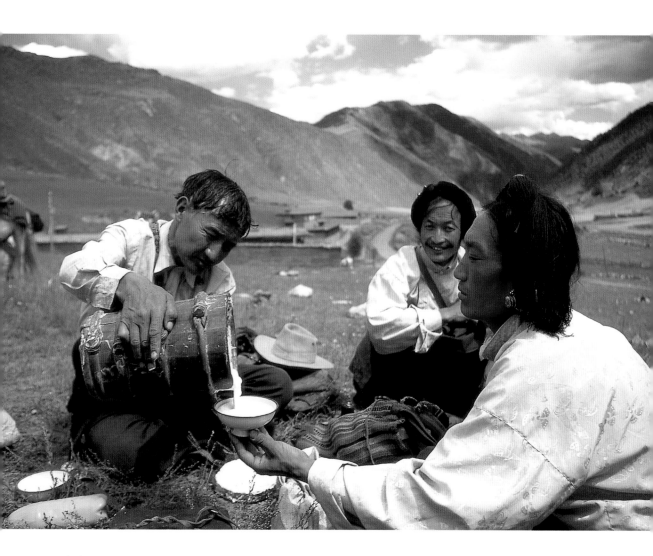

A daily bowel movement is thought to be vital to the digestive process. Your doctor might suggest that you drink some tepid water first thing in the morning and wait for an eliminatory movement within 20 minutes. If you suffer from constipation, you might be advised to take a dessertspoonful of psyllium husks mixed with water each day or to consider colonic irrigation (see page 112).

The disadvantages of dieting

Dieting (in particular a fasting diet) is not practised in Tibetan medicine. Fasting is thought to cause *lung* energy to rise in the body, leading to mental and physical disturbances. The best way to lose weight effectively and permanently is to eat a well-balanced diet that includes plenty of

Mentioned in the Gyud Zhi, *milk is sourced in Tibet from* dri *or female bovines (yaks are the male bovines).*

fresh vegetables and fruit. Traditionally, Tibetan doctors advise taking honey each morning, dissolved in hot or tepid water for those who wish to lose weight, and in hot milk for those who wish to put on weight.

Fasting should also be avoided because food has medicinal properties. This was recognized by the Chinese doctor, Sun Ssu-mo, who wrote in *Prescriptions Worth a Thousand Gold*:

> 'A truly good physician first finds out the cause of the illness, and having found that, he first tries to cure it with food. Only when food fails does he prescribe medication.'

Adapting the Tibetan diet

The staple diet of mainland Tibetans was traditionally — and to a certain extent still is — milk, tsampa (roasted barley), meat (particularly from yaks and sheep) and butter, as found in the infamous salty Tibetan butter tea. These foods are readily obtainable from the harsh environment of Tibet, which, with its high altitude, unforgiving terrain and severe winters, does not permit the cultivation of many vegetables. Barley is both drought- and cold-resistant, which is why it is so prized by the Tibetan people, and alongside meat it enables humankind to survive that land's harsh climate.

Preservation of Tibetan culture

Tibetans say that their cuisine left Tibet when the Dalai Lama went into exile in 1959, taking with him many noble families as well as their cooks and recipes, among them some of the country's best. Tibetan restaurants around the world play an important role in preserving the culture of Tibet. The spicy and innovative cuisine includes ginger with mint sauce used as a table condiment, *momos*, meat-filled dumplings, and noodle broths cooked with garlic and onions. *Thenthuck* soups with dumplings are typical dishes of the community in exile.

Adapting the traditional diet

Today, many Tibetans living in Tibet eat rice as a component of their staple diet, and turnips, potatoes and cabbage feature increasingly on Tibetan dinner tables. Vegetables are readily available in Lhasa's market stalls, which may even have melons for sale. And where once this land-locked country shunned the outside world, it now has difficulty in supplying the demand for fish in its capital.

In recent years the Tibetan diaspora, who live in exile across India and the globe, have found that the traditional high-fat, high-sugar diet that ensured survival in high altitudes is leading in gentler climates to health problems, especially diabetes, high blood pressure and heart disease. Their challenge is to adapt a traditional diet to suit modern ways of living.

Pure food

Food was pure for thousands of years in Tibet, grown in soil and water unpolluted by modern agrichemicals. Today, the nearest we can draw to this ideal is organic food that is produced without the use of artificial pesticides, herbicides, fertilizers or genetically modified organisms, and is inspected regularly to ensure that it meets certification standards. An organic diet benefits not only the environment, wildlife and livestock, but also the health of those who grow and consume the food. A 2001 review of studies from around the world revealed that organic crops have statistically significant higher levels of vitamin C, magnesium, iron, phosphorus and cell-repairing antioxidants than their conventionally grown equivalents. Organic spinach, lettuce, cabbage and potatoes were found to have particularly high levels of minerals.

The principles of good eating

Although a literal interpretation of the traditional Tibetan diet may not be well suited to a modern lifestyle, we can still draw on the principles of eating that were laid out in the Tibetan medical texts, in particular ideas about eating pure food in accordance with the needs of your constitution (see page 92) and the season (see page 98).

In the past, butter made from dri *milk was a vital source of energy in the challenging high-altitude terrain of Tibet.*

The *tantras* discuss food in five groups: grains, oils, meat, liquids, and fruit and vegetables. The following pages explore healthy choices within these groups, bearing in mind the wide range of products that is available to us today. Knowing how these foods affect the body will help you improve your health and reverse disease. Perhaps the most health-giving choice we can make is to avoid ready-prepared meals and instead cook more dishes from scratch and with love, using fresh, organic ingredients.

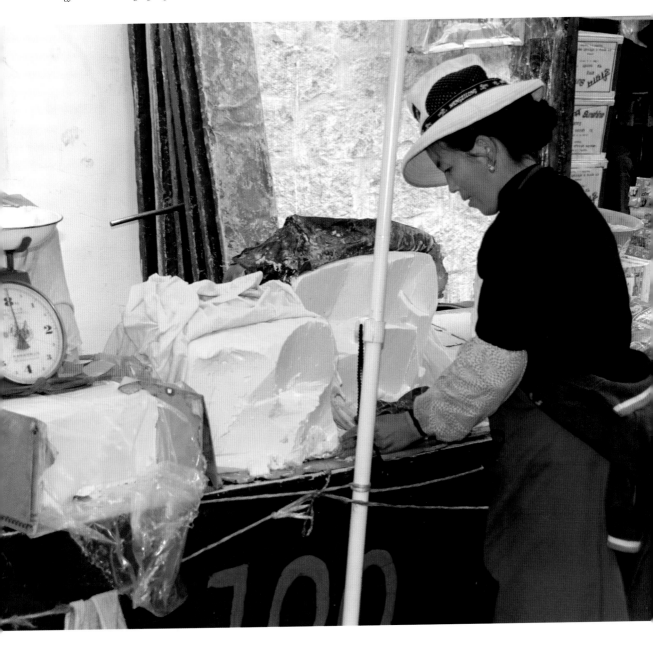

Tibetan food group 1: grains

Grains (or seeds) are of two types: those with pods, such as peas and other pulses, and cereal grains, such as wheat, usually from grasses.

Barley

Tibetans value barley and its strength-giving properties. This grain was, and still is, the staple food of Tibet. High in selenium, phosphorus, copper and manganese, it is also a good source of niacin (vitamin B3) and insoluble fibre, both of which are effective in reducing raised cholesterol levels. Barley can be introduced to a Western diet through soups, casseroles and stews. Steep in water overnight before use.

Rice

Tibetan medicine believes that rice balances all three life forces, increasing vitality and healing digestive upsets. Brown rice, which undergoes less processing than white rice, is by far the most nutritious choice. If this is too much for your palate, American easy-cook rice retains its vitamins well when cooked.

Rice is particularly effective in restoring balance among the three energies, lung, tripa *and* bekan.

Oats

This grain has a long history of use by herbalists as a nerve tonic. Oatmeal is rich in fibre, protein and calcium. Eating just half a cup a day has been proven to reduce cholesterol and strengthen the white blood cells called glucans, bolstering immune function. A study published in the *American Journal of Public Health* found that eating oatmeal regularly could help reduce the risk of adult-onset (or Type-2) diabetes. Add oats to muesli mixes and smoothies, or serve porridge for breakfast.

Quinoa

The United Nations has classified quinoa as a supercrop for its high protein content (12–18 per cent). Unlike the protein in most cereal grains, quinoa protein offers a more complete range of essential amino acids. Known as 'energy porridge' for the rich amount of energy it imparts to the body, quinoa is also a good source of magnesium and iron. Being gluten-free, this grain suits those who cannot tolerate wheat and other grains containing gluten. Use it in salads.

Oats are a nutritious grain, bringing fibre, protein and calcium to the diet.

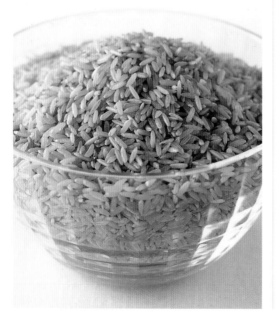

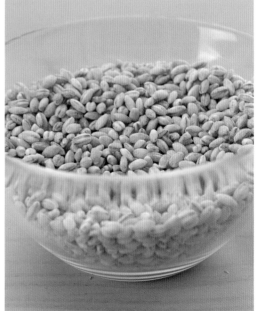

Wheatgerm

This is the part of the wheat seed that provides the nutrients for the successful germination of the shoot. As a result, there are more nutrients per ounce in wheatgerm than in any other grain or vegetable. Rich in fatty acids and proteins, wheatgerm is also a renowned power food. Weight for weight, 100 g (3½ oz) wheatgerm provides more protein than meat. Wheatgerm is also rich in iron and potassium. Sprinkle a little onto breakfast cereal each morning.

Tibetan food group 2: oils

All oils have a sweet taste and restore vitality to the body. They are particularly beneficial for the aged and the young. Tibetans value butter so much that they drink melted butter at night in cupfuls, as it is believed to be a healing panacea. Essential fatty acids are 'essential' because the body cannot produce them, and one of the best sources is oil. For healthy functioning, the brain (which is two-thirds fatty acids) requires a 1:1 ratio of omega-6 essential fatty acids (which are used by the body to produce prostaglandins) to omega-3s (used for normal growth and brain development in children and to protect against heart disease and cancer in adults). As we eat a great deal of processed food in the West, we tend to consume 10–20 times more omega-6 fats than omega-3s. Scientists have made a direct link between high consumption of omega-6 fats/low consumption of omega-3 fats and disease – in particular with mental illness including depression and inflammatory diseases. To redress this imbalance, try to use olive oil, which is an excellent source of monounsaturated omega-9 fatty acids (which help prevent coronary heart disease), or walnut, rapeseed and soya oil, which are high in omega-3 fats.

Sesame oil

This is widely used by Tibetans in cooking and for massage, especially in Ayurvedic massages and hot-oil treatments. This oil is about 47 per cent monounsaturated oleic acid and 39 per cent

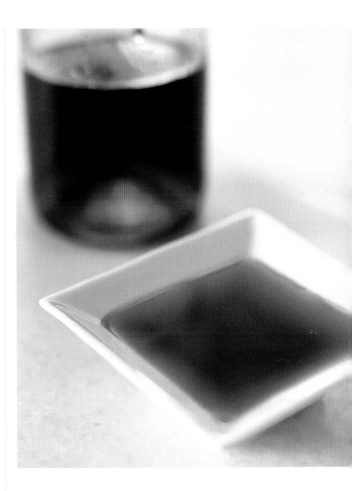

Sesame oil has both nutritional and therapeutic value. Used as a massage oil, it counteracts an excess of lung energy.

linoleic acid (another name for omega-3). A 2005 report by the Agency for Healthcare Research and Quality in Rockville, Maryland, showed that its use helped stop malignant melanoma growth. Westerners should consume sesame oil as it helps to counter stress. It is also very beneficial used as a massage oil, because it pacifies *lung*. Choose organic sesame oil if possible.

Flaxseed oil

More than 50 per cent of this oil comprises omega-3 fatty acids. A dessertspoonful taken daily in the morning is a sufficient supplement to your diet. Flaxseed or linseed oil must be consumed when it is very fresh, and kept refrigerated. Add it to salads, in a ratio of one part flaxseed oil to ten parts olive oil.

Tibetan food group 3: meat

According to the medical *tantras*, meats have a sweet post-digestive aftertaste. Fresh meat is cooling, while dried meat combats diseases associated with *lung*. Meat from birds of prey is believed to disperse tumours.

If you live in the West, it is best to eat organic meat from animals that have been reared without pesticides and antibiotics and have been more humanely treated. Cattle and sheep produce a large amount of methane, a greenhouse gas that contributes to global warming. It is therefore a good idea to try to reduce your consumption of red meat, which has in any case been shown to increase the risk of cancer.

Tibetan food group 4: liquids

Liquids are essential for health and water in particular is needed by the body for all its biological processes. Many Westerners do not drink sufficient water and are dehydrated. Liquids such as fresh milk are a source of essential vitamins and some minerals.

Milk

The milk referred to in the *Gyud Zhi* is fresh, unprocessed milk sourced from the *dri* (female counterpart of the yak). Tibetans have reared these bovine animals for centuries, as (unlike crops) they enable a traditional nomadic lifestyle.

Most of the milk consumed in the West is from intensively reared cattle treated with antibiotics and hormones, and has been pasteurized (which denatures its nutrients through heating) and homogenized (a process that may make it harder to digest). Some people choose to consume instead local untreated milk or milk from organically reared cows. A 2006 study showed organic milk to be 68 per cent higher in omega-3 fatty acids than milk from standard dairy cows.

Some people find goat's milk the most digestible. Unsweetened natural or 'live' yogurt is also beneficial because its active culture of bacteria, *lactobacillus*, helps to fortify the immune system. Colostrum– the first milk provided for the young calf – is so rich in active immune components that it is known as 'nature's antibiotic' and is available as dried tablets. Studies in sports science show that bovine colostrum can promote natural muscle growth, and is effective against irritable bowel syndrome, leaky gut and chronic fatigue syndrome.

A glass of wine taken with food each day can protect against heart disease and provide the antioxidant resveratrol.

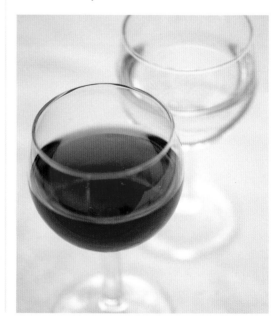

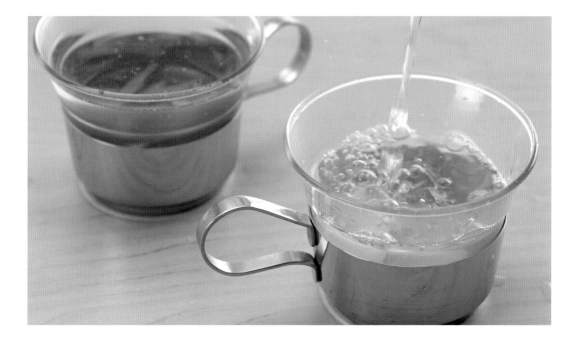

Ginger tea restores fire to your digestive system and is especially valuable for sluggish bekan *types.*

Wheatgrass juice

This bright-green juice is a complete food, containing enzymes, vitamins, 17 amino acids, 92 minerals and chlorophyll. It contains 18 times more iron than a comparable quantity of spinach and more vitamin A than carrots. Juiced, 454 g (1 lb) of wheatgrass is equivalent in nutritional value to 10 kg (23 lb) of garden vegetables. Wheatgrass may offer protection against dietary carcinogens and is said to be unique in dissolving scar tissue in the lungs, detoxifying the body, cleaning the blood and buffering corrosive acids. Its enzymes are even said to dissolve tumours. Try a 25 ml (1 fl oz) shot daily or weekly.

Wine

In Tibet, *chang*, brewed from fermented barley, is the beer most commonly drunk on religious days and offered to deities. In the West, wine taken in moderation is a good substitute. A long tradition of using wine medicinally stretches back to Hippocrates (460–377 BCE), the Greek physician often considered the 'father of medicine', and Paracelsus (1493–1541), the father of modern pharmacology, who extolled the health-giving properties of wine. Many vineyards are close to monasteries that used to cultivate grapes to make wine for medicinal and sacramental use.

Wine can be a rich source of easily digestible minerals, antioxidant polyphenols (five times more powerful than vitamin E), and anticoagulant and relaxant ingredients. Studies have shown that responsible wine drinkers are less likely to develop heart and neuro-degenerative disease than teetotallers. Wine also seems to improve osteoporosis and macular degeneration, as well as digestive problems, from indigestion to constipation. The valuable antioxidant in wine – resveratrol – even seems to activate DNA repair. A glass of wine drunk with food is the best way to include it in your daily diet.

Tea

Tibetans traditionally drink salty butter tea, an energy-giving beverage suitable for high altitudes. For those living Western lifestyles, herbal teas make a great alternative to caffeine drinks and a convenient way of ingesting healing herbs. Place herbs such as camomile, liquorice or cardamom seeds to cover the bottom of a cup, pour over boiling water and leave to infuse before sipping.

Tibetan food group 5: fruit and vegetables

This category includes both vegetables and fruit and just a few of the most valuable examples are described below. In general, we need to be eating as many greens as possible to counteract the health problems, such as cancer, heart disease and diabetes, which are associated with a typical Western diet that is high in animal fats and processed foods. Green vegetables contain many cancer-fighting phytochemicals. To take just one example, broccoli contains sulphoraphane, which activates a group of enzymes that literally soak up carcinogens from the cells.

Fruit

Like other foods in Tibetan medicine, fruits are described according to their taste and potency: bananas are sweet-tasting but heavy and oily in their effect on the constitution; oranges are sour and sweet, and have a light and cooling effect.

Fruits are best eaten in the morning, as they have a detoxifying effect on the body. Prioritize bitartrate fruits, such as yellow grapefruit, lemons and limes, which – contrary to popular belief – have an alkalizing effect when ingested and can therefore help to maintain optimum blood pH levels. To detoxify the liver, drink yellow grapefruit juice. For a complete body detoxification, eat red grapes. Fresh pineapple is particularly beneficial for body maintenance and repair since it contains the anti-inflammatory enzyme bromelain. (Some naturopaths suggest that patients take bromelain before and after surgery to speed the healing process.) The enzyme also helps asthma sufferers as it reduces the inflammation that can trigger an attack.

To ensure you are getting enough vitamin C from natural food in winter, consume frozen fruits and berries, which have high levels of antioxidants. In the West, oranges and other citrus fruits are also excellent sources of vitamin C and other antioxidants.

Tibetan goji berries

These berries contain significant levels of antioxidants, over 500 times more vitamin C than oranges and large amounts of the cancer-protection minerals selenium and germanium. Goji berries can be bought from supermarkets. Alternatively, visit the website of the Tanaduk Botanical Research Institute, an organization that cultivates and preserves Tibetan medicinal plants. Use goji berries in stir-fries or sprinkled on breakfast cereal or salads, or soak them and juice them or make them into jam.

Avocados

Easily digestible, high in monounsaturated fats and containing vitamins A, B and E as well as 17 minerals, avocados are a total food. They have a lower sugar content than bananas but a higher content of potassium, which may help to avert hypertension (increased potassium levels are associated with decreased blood pressure). In a study published in the *Journal of Nutritional Biochemistry*, an extract of avocado was found to inhibit the growth of prostate cancer cells. Enjoy a few slices in a tossed salad, or spread on bread instead of butter.

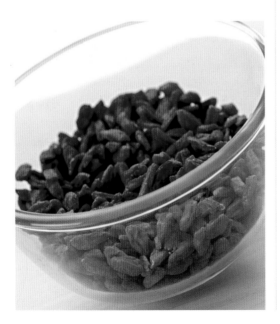

Tibetan goji berries contain 500 times more vitamin C than oranges, as well as high levels of selenium and germanium.

Tomatoes

Rich in the biochemical lycopene, which has been found to reduce the risk of prostate cancer, tomatoes also contain coumaric acid and chlorogenic acid, which may block the effect of suspected carcinogenic nitrosamines. Tomatoes are also a good source of vitamin A, vitamin C and potassium. A study undertaken by Harvard Medical School of 48,000 men found that those who ate ten or more servings of tomato products a week had a 35 per cent lower risk of prostate cancer than those who did not. Try to include concentrated and cooked tomato products in your diet, as these are 400 per cent higher in lycopene than fresh tomatoes.

Sprouted seeds and beans

Seeds and beans contain within them all the vitamins, proteins and fats required to ensure germination. When sprouted, they may be considered a 'living food'. The biochemical process of sprouting transforms proteins into easily absorbed simple amino acids, increases the levels of vitamin C, folic acid and vitamin B6, and processes minerals into a form that the body can utilize. Sprouts are also full of antioxidants – broccoli sprouts have been found to have more than 50 times the antioxidant sulphoraphane than does mature broccoli. A University of Ulster study found that eating 100 g (3½ oz) of sprouts a day for two weeks protected blood cells from DNA damage. Possibilities for sprouting include chickpeas, linseeds, peanuts, alfalfa, broccoli, sunflower seeds and buckwheat.

Soya

One of the main dietary sources of the plant hormones isoflavones is soya. Structurally, isoflavones are similar to human oestrogens, but they are much less active at the body's oestrogen receptor sites. As a result, they can reduce high oestrogen levels by ousting the stronger natural oestrogens at the oestrogen receptors. They are also thought to block the take-up by oestrogen receptors of pesticides, which mimic oestrogen

'Let your food be your medicine and your medicine be your food'

Hippocrates

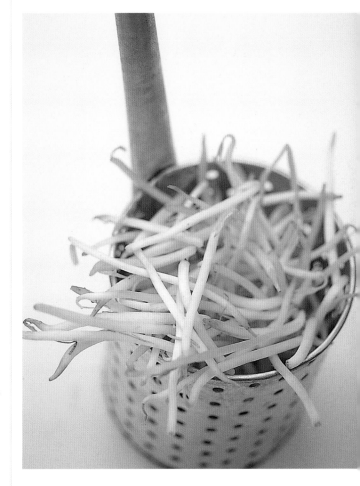

Traditionally used in Asian cookery, bean sprouts are a 'living food' packed full of vitamins and antioxidants.

in the body and have been linked to cancer. Studies attribute a lack of menopausal symptoms in Japan and a low incidence of breast cancer in Chinese women to high blood levels of phyto-oestrogens resulting from a high consumption of soya. Soya milk is also a good replacement for dairy milk if you are lactose intolerant.

Living with your constitution

After a doctor of Tibetan medicine has diagnosed your constitutional or nyepa *type as primarily* lung, tripa *or* bekan *(see page 53), try to follow a diet that will keep these three internal life energies in balance. Eating according to your type is an important part of Tibetan medicine and a means of promoting good health.*

Eating for your *nyepa* type

Tibetan medicine approaches diet with an awareness of the effects of heating and cooling foods. In choosing and cooking food, the aim is to avoid aggravating the harmony of the three energies. Remember that dieting is frowned upon in Tibetan medicine, especially for *lung* types, as it exacerbates their constitution.

Lung types

The word *lung* relates to 'winds' and the nervous system. *Lung* types should eat a diet that is high in protein and take three regular meals a day. Breakfast is important because it grounds those with excessive *lung* energy. A protein drink should set you up for the day. Don't leave your main meal until late in the day, or you may feel sluggish and then be unable to sleep. Eating late will also impact on your liver, making it hard for you to get up the next morning.

Sweet, sour and salty foods (such as custard with honey, chutney and ham) are best for *lung* types as they increase internal body warmth, which is beneficial for someone with lots of *lung* energy. To keep the energies in balance, eat porridge and muesli for breakfast, meat soups with nutmeg and oily main courses that include items such as avocados, vegetables roasted in oil and bean casserole. Add some sesame oil to soups and stews.

Foods that *lung* types eat should be cooked or warmed first. Stewed fruits such as rhubarb and apple with cinnamon are good, while raw fruit, cold desserts, ice creams, caffeine drinks,

Include nutmeg in the diet if you are a lung *type or you are suffering from an excess of* lung *energy.*

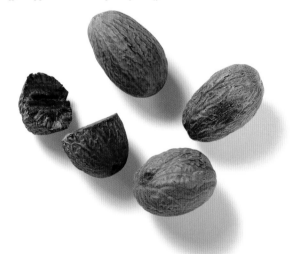

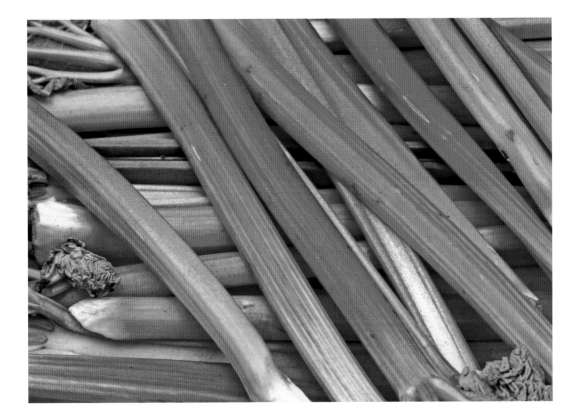

convenience foods, potatoes and a diet containing lots of salad are best avoided.

When *lung* is out of balance or in excess, include nutmeg in the diet as much as possible, and eat oily and moistening foods, such as thick, brothy soups containing sesame or olive oil or meat casseroles cooked with butter.

Tripa types

The word *tripa* means 'heat' and relates to body temperature and metabolism. *Tripa* types should eat foods that are sweet, astringent and bitter. Astringent foods like garlic cause the channels to contract, helping the energies to remain in their location in the body, while bitter foods like lemon and various herbs stimulate the stomach to produce digestive juices. Foods that cause internal heat, such as lamb, curries and spicy indigenous foods, are best avoided. Vegetables should be eaten raw as often as possible, as well as cold tofu, salads and sprouted grains, which are very rich in nutrients. Fresh raw juices are excellent for the *tripa* type. *Tripa* excess of heat is

If you are a lung *type, stewed fruit such as rhubarb is preferable to fruit eaten raw.*

Cold tofu is excellent for the tripa *type, who should aim to include cooling foods in the diet.*

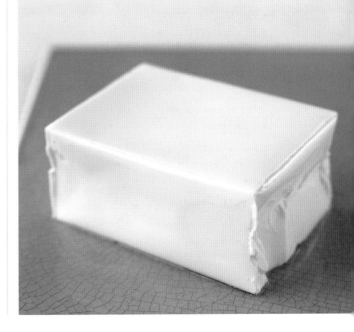

often seen in the form of gas and acid in the stomach. When this happens you can cool the body down with foods such as fresh juices and live yogurt. Flatulence may also be due to stress, which can lead to an imbalance of gut bacteria. Taking probiotic supplements or live yogurt is an excellent remedy in this case.

Tripa types can include some spice in the diet, but this should be mainly confined to coriander, which can have a cooling effect on the body. Avoid any hot spices like chillies, which may aggravate a *tripa* constitution. Breakfast could consist of yellow grapefruit or lemon juice and yogurt with honey; lunch of a salad, such as mixed bean salad with turmeric rice or salmon with a mixed-leaf salad and lime dressing; and the evening meal of chicken or fish with leafy vegetables and rice.

Garlic helps contract the energy channels, which is beneficial for both tripa *and* bekan *types.*

Bekan types

Bekan relates to body fluids and lubrication. *Bekan* types feel the cold, so they need heating foods with a 'kick' to get them going (they love their rest!). They should eat warm foods that are easy to digest, with lunch being the most important meal. A little gentle exercise after the meal aids digestion and the flow of internal energies.

Breakfast could include pancakes with honey and a hot drink of fresh ginger or chai tea, and a protein milkshake or some Greek yogurt may suffice for lunch. Astringent garlic helps the channels to contract, beneficial for *bekan* types as for *tripa* types. Rich curries are good for *bekan* types, keeping them warm; chillies can also be added to food. For an evening meal, something like couscous, quinoa or rice with chickpeas or lentils, or a lamb curry, will satisfy the appetite.

Adding chillies during cooking is a simple way of achieving the heating foods that benefit bekan *constitutional types.*

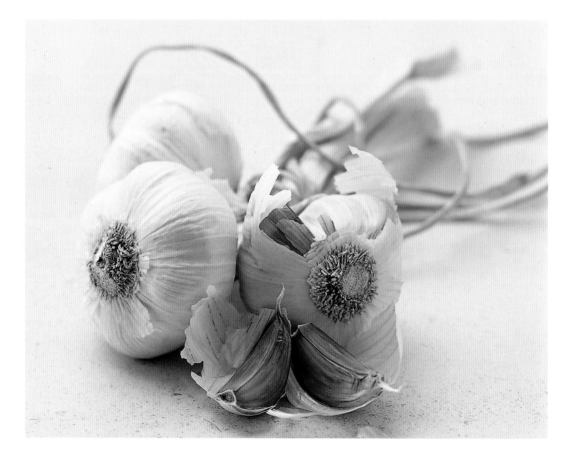

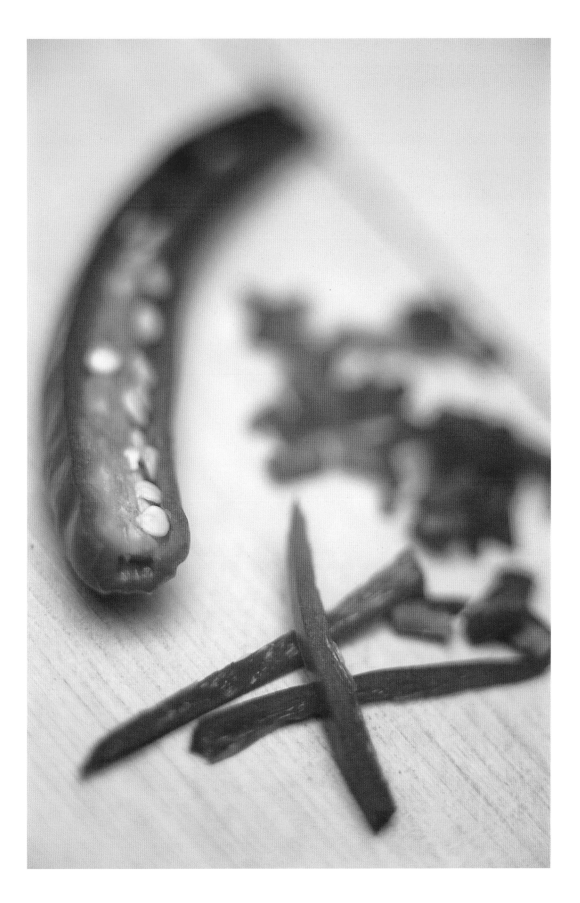

Living with the seasons

The seasons are the clock of nature, marking how the natural world dies and renews itself every 12 months. As without, so within: your entire body and its cells and organs are also in a state of constant renewal, just like nature's cycle of death and rebirth. And just as the tides of our oceans are influenced by the gravitational pull of the moon, so too is the internal energetic that the Tibetans call la, *which travels around the body and reaches the crown chakra every full moon.*

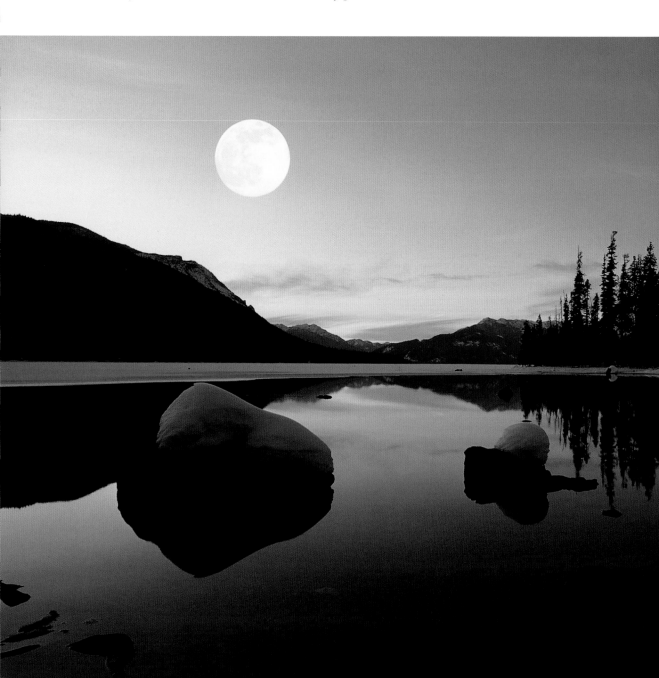

The energies of the planet

The movement of the seasons causes nature's animals to hibernate and mate and its flowers to bloom. The energies of the natural world and its five elements of earth, water, fire, air and space likewise cause us to sleep at night and to grow, and our metabolisms to increase and decrease. In Western science these cyclical changes are described as 'biorhythms'.

Practising the art of healing in harmony with the energies of the planet is fundamental to Tibetan medicine, which must be applied with an understanding of these forces and of the seasons. The universal life force, manifesting in the body as the divine consciousness *tsog-lung*, produces the seven bodily constituents: nutritional essence, blood, flesh, fat, bone, marrow and regenerative fluid. These processes occur within a universal matrix of the five elements and in the specific seasonal context. According to the medical *tantras*, disease may manifest, increase and subside due to the energies of the seasons.

Solar energy and the solstices

As solar energy becomes stronger in our planet, the mountain ice peaks begin to melt, as do the polar ice caps. Similarly, the phlegm in the body starts to melt from winter onwards and in spring phlegmatic conditions proliferate. Tibetan medicine recommends washing with a mixture of lentil flour and soap powder, instead of soap, to remove excess phlegm from the body. To disperse phlegm in early spring, you should also start yoga exercises or – if you are a practitioner of Buddha *Dharma* – begin prostrations to the Buddhas and deities (see page 138).

During the summer, when the fire element is at its greatest, heating activities such as saunas should be avoided. Meditation is important at this time. If you can, meditate outdoors during summer evenings. Meditating into the blue sky

The moon influences the passage of the life force la *around the body's chakras, both following the same 28-day cycle.*

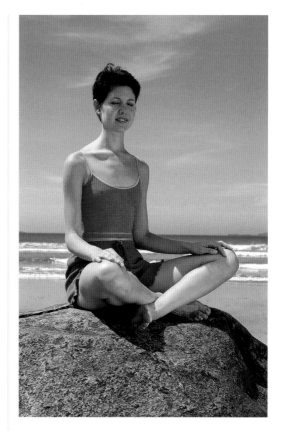

In the summer, try to meditate outside as much as possible, letting your troubles float away into the clear blue sky.

with the sun behind you for 20 minutes will allow you to release the stress of the day into the vastnesses of the sky and relax your mind.

Tibetan medicine and the practice of Tantric Buddhism pay particular attention to the spring and summer solstice. As the sun moves northwards on the spring solstice fire energy begins to grow, heating the planet and giving people their strength. At the winter solstice fire energy peaks and at this point the sun starts its descent again and the lunar energies that are cooler become predominant.

Bekan types in particular need to start getting fit in early spring to get their metabolism going. From the time of the spring equinox until the winter equinox, all physical types should make the most of their increased energy. Tibetan medicine also recommends reducing excessive sexual activity at this time. Some may even want to refrain from sex for certain periods. In particular, men are advised to be careful of ejaculation, as losing ejaculate means losing life essence. (By eating foods like oysters at this time they can replace zinc lost through ejaculate.)

The heat of summer will exacerbate the *tripa* energy present in *tripa* types. It is a good idea for them to take up regular swimming during the hot months, to calm the imbalance of this energy.

Tibetan medicine teaches that, from the time of the autumn equinox, all the constitutional types can have as much sex as they like. Sex is considered especially useful for people in whom *lung* energy predominates, because it alleviates the stress they are prone to accumulating.

Suppression of bodily functions is discouraged in the medical *tantras*. For example, they state that you must eat if you are hungry and that you can create kidney stones by not urinating. You must not hold your breath for prolonged periods, because holding the breath regularly under exertion is said to bring about heart disease.

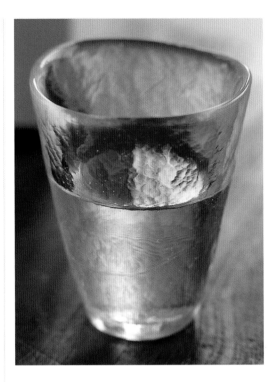

Drink plenty of water from a pure source during the summer months to avoid dehydration.

Diet and the seasons

In spring, bitter, spicy and sour foods should be eaten to keep phlegm diseases from rising. Lemon, ginger and stewed apples are good examples of these. Water boiled with honey should also be taken. If you are naturally phlegmatic you can take an emetic in the early spring to release accumulated phlegm.

In summer, all constitutional types should avoid heating foods, such as curries, casseroles made with lamb and hot spices. Veer towards salads during this season, with protein in forms such as organic goat's cheese or raw tofu. Drink chilled white wine or beer, but in moderation with lots of ice. Most importantly, drink plenty of water to avoid becoming dehydrated.

In autumn, all constitutional types should eat more of the foods that foster internal heat. Choose apples instead of lemons, for example,

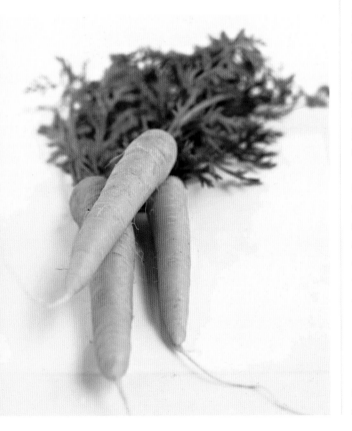

Eat root vegetables, such as carrots, in autumn because they are both warming foods and seasonal at this time.

and instead of salads eat root vegetables such as carrots, parsnips, aubergines and butternut squash, roasted or made into soups.

As autumn moves into winter, your appetite will increase and you can eat as much as you like of the warming foods. Avoid the foods that foster internal cooling, such as salads, uncooked tofu and cold drinks.

Protecting against disease

Disease comes to dirty places, so keeping your home clean and the air as fresh as possible, by daily airing of the house, will offer protection. If you do not want to open the windows during the coldest months, you should burn healing Tibetan incense. This may be sourced through the website of the Mentseekhang.

During spring and summer, you can spray essential oils diluted with water around your

Burning healing incense during autumn and winter will clear the air and protect your home from disease.

'The power of plants and plant extracts should never be underestimated'

home. Lemongrass has been found to be an excellent deodorizer and geranium is good for balance and harmony. A few drops of each essential oil in some water will suffice. Tea-tree oil is a powerful antiseptic, used for example by the Australian armed forces during the Second World War. The power of plants and plant extracts should never be underestimated.

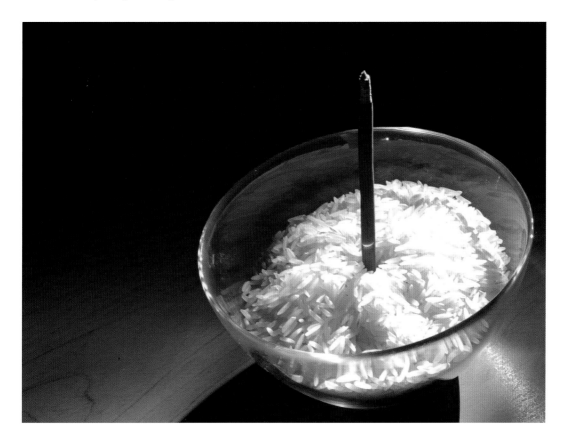

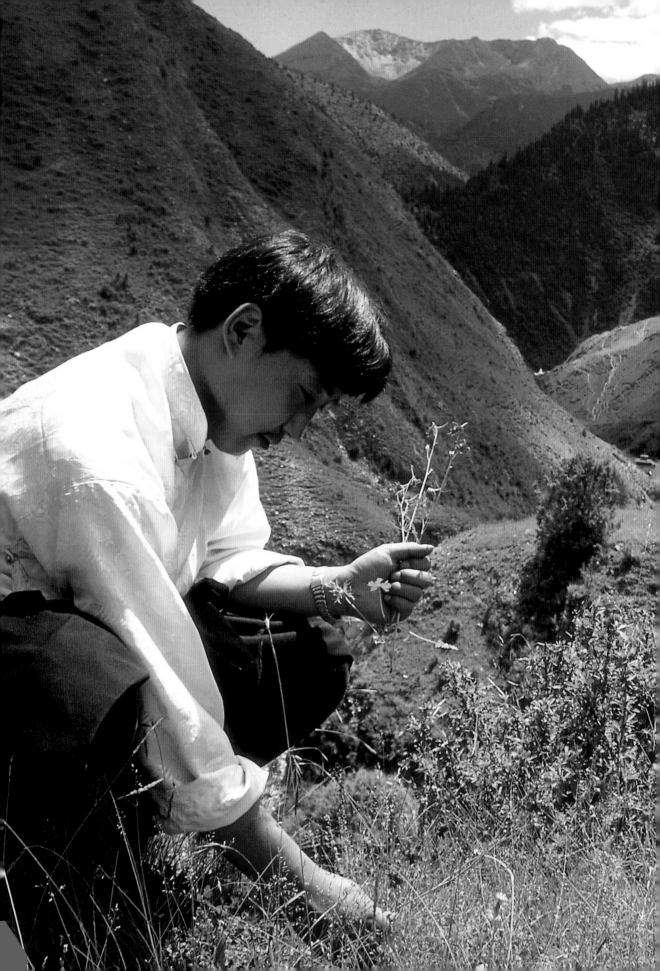

Therapeutic remedies

Achieving homeostasis or mental and physical harmony of the entire organism is the goal of Tibetan medicine, not the temporary relief of symptoms. If changes to diet and lifestyle fail to bring this about, Tibetan doctors turn to herbal formulas, which they have traditionally gathered and manufactured themselves. They know the effects of more than 1,000 herbs in many combinations. The next option for treatment is hands-on therapies, such as moxibustion or cupping, which stimulate energy points on the body. Another option open to doctors is to prescribe the pills created by spiritual masters according to secret formulas through profound alchemical processes.

Tibetan herbal medicine

After addressing diet and behavioural changes, herbal formulas are the first remedies to which doctors of Tibetan medicine turn in order to restore balance to the three life energies within the body. Tibetan doctors are expert pharmacists who never prescribe single herbs. Healing plants are only ever given in synergy and some of the thousands of formulas are very complex. Each pill can contain anything from seven to 100 ingredients, and so over the centuries a large materia medica, or compilation of therapeutic remedies, has been built up through the practice of herbal medicine.

The materia medica

The current materia medica of Tibet is derived from *The Pearl Herbs* (*Jingzhu Bencao*), which was published in 1835 by Dumar Danzhenpengcuo. The text is made up of two sections, one composed of *sutra* praise and the other classifying the raw materials that can be used to create healing remedies. According to the medical *tantras*, everything on earth has the power to be a medicine. *The Pearl Herbs* lists 2,294 materials, of which 1,006 are of plant origin, 448 of animal origin and 840 are minerals. Today, animal materials are no longer used, and more than 300 of Tibet's medicinal plants have become extinct since the Chinese invasion.

Herbal formulas

Although the herbs are described individually, they are never used alone in Tibetan herbal remedies, but instead are used in synergistic combinations that are designed to regulate the effects of the active ingredients on the body. It has been observed that the side-effects commonly experienced with Western pharmaceutical medicine are not observed in Tibetan medicine, and this may be attributed to the complexity of the herbal formulas.

Divinely revealed healing

All the healing plants in the world are believed to have been planted by the healing female medicine deity known as Yitrogma. Before the advent of modern research techniques, shamans and herbalists across the world relied on two broad laws to determine which plants had uses as a herbal medicine. The first is called the 'doctrine of contraries', in which balance is sought by countering one quality with its opposite (such as the use of cooling herbs to treat fevers).

The second philosophy is the 'doctrine of signatures', which taught that like cured like: a plant's shape gave a clue to the parts of the body with which it had an affinity (for example, pilewort looks like piles and treats them effectively). Healers would also watch sick animals and note what they ate to heal themselves. Many of the healing properties attributed to plants using these doctrines have now been scientifically proven to have that healing effect.

Because much of Tibet was shamanistic in nature before the arrival of Buddhism in the 7th century, part of the materia medica may have been found by shamans during mystical trance states, perhaps provoked using ethnogens,

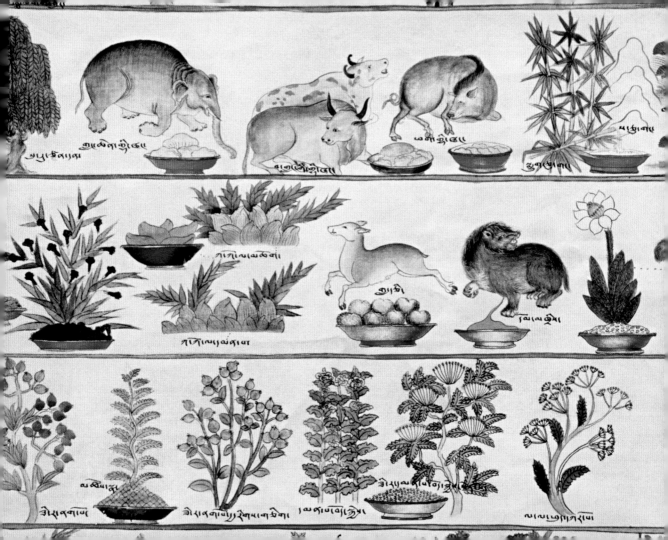

psychedelically active substances. During these trances the spirits of the forest would instruct the shaman on which herbs should be used in the treatment of disease.

Tibetan doctors, who are considered to be emanations of the Medicine Buddha, sometimes dream of patients before they meet them. The healing angels of the Medicine Buddha help the doctors towards a diagnosis and instruct them on which herbs might effect a lasting cure. Doctors are also said to have sometimes sourced herbs and healing formulas from them.

The inhabitants of Tibet see the natural world as their medicine cabinet. Here, a cure for toothache is prepared.

Secret knowledge

Many books on Tibetan herbal medicine have not yet been translated from their original language. Translation is made difficult because some of the words used are secret synonyms. The term 'myrobalan', for example, has 32 synonyms in Tibetan and 42 in Sanskrit.

The make-up of the herbal formulas is so closely guarded that the preparation of medicines is passed from a Tibetan doctor of the lineage of Tantric healers only to his close disciples. Many formulas are stored in a cryptic form to safeguard their contents from charlatans and can only be deciphered after the oral transmission of a bona fide master of healing.

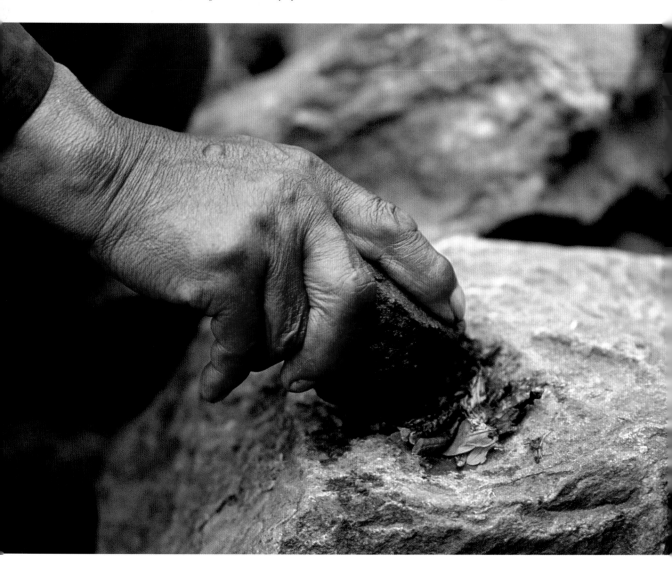

Herbal training

To train to become a master pharmacist of Tibetan medicine takes at least seven years. A trainee must learn the properties of each of the herbs in the pharmacopoeia, and where and how to gather them. A pharmacist is also trained in the medicinal 'tastes' of the herbs and their effects within the body. All Tibetan doctors are required to study herbal pharmacy and to learn to make medicines themselves. They are instructed in three aspects in the formulation of herbal pills: balancing, enhancing and protection from side-effects.

Taste, powers and effects

Pharmacists produce Tibetan medicines according to their taste, power and effects, a combination of considerations unique to Tibetan medicine that may perhaps account for its lack of negative side-effects. The six tastes are categorized as sweet, sour, bitter, salty, spicy and astringent. There are also three post-digestive tastes, considered to be sweet, sour and bitter, each of which balances two of the three life forces, *lung, tripa* and *bekan*.

The eight powers have different effects on the internal energies of the body. They are categorized as heavy, smooth, cool, soft, light, rough, spicy and sharp.

The 17 effects are approached by doctors with the understanding that a cold disease is healed by a hot effect, a damp condition is healed by a dry effect, and so on. The effects are categorized as follows: cold, hot, warm, cool, thick, thin, moist, rough, light, heavy, steady, motive, blunt, sharp, tender, dry and soft. By considering all of the above in the formulation of medicine, a Tibetan doctor works in harmony with nature and its five elements, as they manifest both externally to the body and internally.

Pacification and elimination

The *Gyud Zhi* describes the power of Tibetan herbal medicine as having two aspects: pacifying and eliminating. Pacifying medicines subdue an excess of a particular vital energy, encouraging it

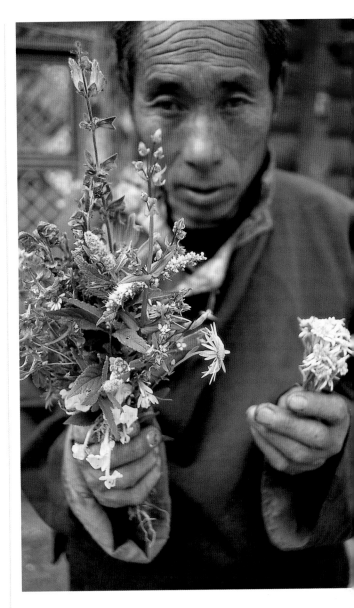

These medicinal plants may be used for the cure of foot and mouth disease in animals, known as kasha *in Tibetan.*

back to its correct location in the body. These include a Tibetan medicine known as Agar, which encourages *lung* energy to balance and return to its proper location.

Eliminating medicines are prescribed to expel excessive amounts of a vital force from the body and to cleanse the mystical channels through which it flows. These types of medicine and treatments include suppositories, enemas, emetics and nasal-cleansing techniques.

The Tibetan pharmacopoeia

Among the items in the Tibetan pharmacopoeia are the herbs and minerals that are depicted being held by the Medicine Buddha in his mandala, referred to as his healing paradise. This is a wonderful pictorial representation of the Tibetan medical pharmacopoeia. Groups of herbs are described as four 'mountains', associated with the four cardinal points of the compass.

East Mountain – supreme medicine

Terminalia chebula, the tree of health, known as myrobalan or arura in Tibetan medicine, is the plant the Medicine Buddha holds in his left hand as a gesture of healing to all who see him. Every part of the myrobalan tree can be used in healing. Uniquely in the natural world, the tree comprises all six tastes, seven powers and 17 effects of Tibetan herbal medicine (see page 105).

The fruits of the tree are seen as particularly special and are believed to promote longevity and wisdom. They function as a nerve tonic, heart calmative and digestive balancer. There is believed to be a form of myrobalan made of gold, but it would be necessary to travel to the Buddha realms to see it.

In his book *Tibetan Buddhist Medicine and Psychiatry*, Terry Clifford describe the power of the myrobalan tree:

> 'The root is good for bone diseases, the trunk for flesh, the branch for nerve disorders and sinew, the bark for skin, the leaf for diseases of the "hollow organs", the flower for the sense organs, and the fruit for the heart and solid organs.'

North Snowclad Mountain – herbs for hot illnesses

Sandalwood, camphor and liquorice are some of the herbs used for cooling hot diseases (see page 69) and are thought to be influenced by the power of the moon. Inflammation, according to Tibetan medicine, creates heat and spreads in the body, causing tissues to become repeatedly inflamed and break down faster than they can be repaired. Western science teaches that most diseases are an inflammatory response to stress and are attempts by the body's biochemistry to repair itself, whereas Tibetans believe that all disease is triggered by stress aggravating *lung*.

South Thunderbolt Mountain – herbs for cold illnesses

Cinnamon, ginger, pomegranate and black pepper are the main herbs of the South Thunderbolt Mountain. They are generally used in the treatment of cold diseases (see page 69), as they are influenced by the power of the sun.

West Malaya Mountain Six Excellent Medicines – *dzang drug*

The six important herbs associated with the West Malaya Mountain are nutmeg, clove, bamboo, saffron, cubeb and cardamom.

Nutmeg (*dzati*)

Both the fruit and oil of this plant are used to combat all types of *lung* disorders. Nutmeg has a direct effect on the *srog rtsa* life channel (see page 48), the seat of consciousness. Its active principle is myristicin, known to be a powerful

This Medicine Buddha mandala depicts myrobalan, clove, pepper and the other main ingredients of Tibetan medicine.

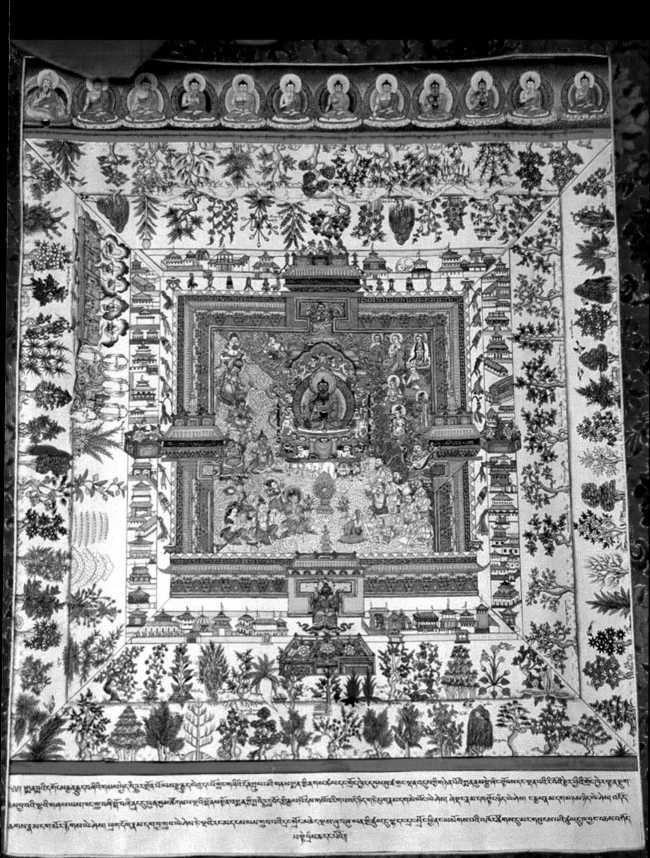

anti-inflammatory, to prevent damage to the bowel by *E. coli* and to inhibit cancer caused by chemical poisoning. It is said that if no other medicine can be found for psychiatric disorders, inhaling nutmeg will suffice. Nutmeg is recommended to pacify disturbance of the winds in the *srog rtsa* channel, which is also why it is used to treat heart disease. The flesh of the nutmeg is shaped like a heart and so nutmeg is also used as a male aphrodisiac.

Clove (*lishi*)

This spice is used to treat the *srog rtsa* channel and, more specifically, the minor channels connected to it. It is traditionally known to be helpful in cases of angina pectoris. This warming herb generates heat and is good in the treatment of cold disorders. The active principle in clove is eugenol, a powerful anaesthetic and bacteria inhibitor, used for centuries in dentistry. The antioxidant effect of its essential oil is the most powerful of all plants.

Bamboo (*chugang*)

The sap of this plant is used to treat phlegm-causing diseases and is rich in silica, a trace element needed by the body to maintain healthy bones and skin. The bamboo sap is effective in breaking up phlegm, especially that which is thought to collect around the heart, causing insomnia and epilepsy. Tradition holds bamboo to be very effective in treating asthma.

Saffron (*khache-gurgum*)

One of the world's most expensive spices, saffron is often used to dye Buddhist robes. This spice also has a lengthy tradition of use in medicine. For example, archeologists have discovered paintings in Greece that depict saffron's use in treating more than 90 diseases. In the Middle East, saffron baths were considered a health panacea. Research has revealed that saffron is rich in vitamin B2 and carotenoids (natural anti-cancer agents) and that it protects the digestive system. Tibetan medicine recognizes it as beneficial for the liver, and it has been used by many cultures to treat depression.

Cubeb (*gurgum*)

In Tibetan medicine this plant is renowned for treatment of the spleen and has a history of treating gonorrhoea and urinary problems such as cystitis. The essential oil is antiseptic and is used in the formulation of throat lozenges.

Cardamom (*sugsmel*)

This queen of spices is used in oriental medicine to dispel damp. It is especially useful in the treatment of stomach complaints, such as acidity and flatulence. It contains the compound cineole, which is a known nerve tonic and antiseptic. This spice is also used to treat impotence. Egyptians used it to whiten teeth, and recent research has proved it to be helpful in dentistry.

Using herbs at home

Healing herbs are an essential part of Tibetan medicine and some of them are probably already in your kitchen cupboard. Once you learn their benefits you can use them in a variety of different ways. Recent scientific studies have shown that some herbs can outperform pharmaceuticals in their curative action, without side-effects.

Herbal baths

One very powerful treatment in Tibetan medicine is herbal bath therapy. Doctors of Tibetan medicine use it particularly in the treatment of arthritis and skin complaints, and the therapy is so successful that they are eager to promote its methods of alleviating pain. Scientific studies have demonstrated the beneficial effects of Tibetan herbal baths on rheumatoid arthritis, finding that the baths decreased the immune system activity that causes the disease.

During the seventh month of the Tibetan calendar (early autumn), a star appears that is associated with the medicine deity Garma Duiba. During this time, Tibetans call any water touched by this starlight 'dew'. The appearance of the star marks the start of the Tibetan bathing festival.

Five Taste Dew is a standard Tibetan bath formula for a healing bath therapy that is practised every day for a minimum of seven days. The formula is made from five herbs: Italian cypress, sweet wormwood, azalea, ephedra and nutmeg. These herbs all have healing qualities.

Italian cypress is a known antiviral and also helps cure skin conditions such as eczema and dermatitis. Sweet wormwood has recently been found to be beneficial in the treatment of malaria: its active compound, artemisinin, has been shown to cut the death rate of those treated with it by 97 per cent. Sweet wormwood has also been shown to help prevent the development of cancer cells. The flowers of red azalea have a detoxifying effect, strengthen the heart and help balance the emotions. Ephedra is great for aches and pains caused by feeling cold, and stimulates sweating. Nutmeg calms the heart and is good for all *lung* disorders.

Use a handful of each herb for each bath, plus one whole nutmeg, grated. (See page 110 for instruction on how to make a herbal bath.)

Massage oils

Massage is therapy widely used in Tibetan medicine to promote the free flow of *tsog-lung* around the body (see page 116). It is easy to make a massage oil using unadulterated organic

You can make an authentic herbal massage oil using a mix of essential oils blended with stress-relieving sesame oil.

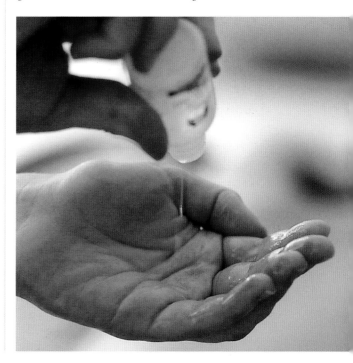

Making a herbal bath

This simple formula for a herbal bath, combining juniper berries, lemon balm, camomile and lavender, is recommended for use during the rejuvenation programme (see page 115)

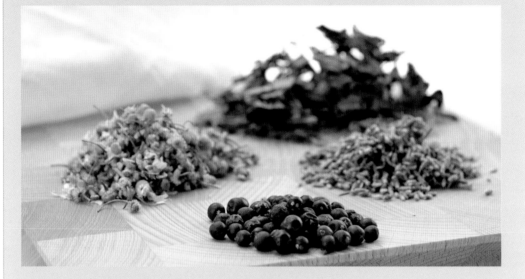

1 You will need a handful each of lemon balm, camomile and lavender, and a tablespoon of juniper seeds.

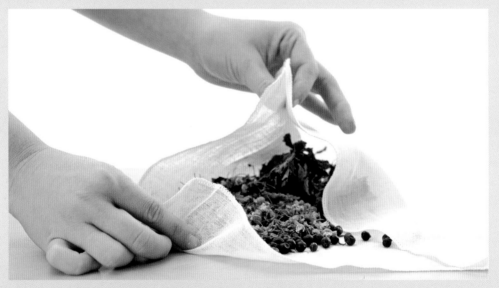

2 Place in a muslin square and tie securely. Leave to steep for about ten minutes and then get in the bath and remain there for at least 20 minutes, relaxing in the water.

essential oils. As your base oil, choose colourless sesame oil, traditionally used to counter stress. To 100 ml (3½ fl oz) of sesame oil, add these essential oils: ten drops of clove, five drops of sandalwood, five drops of cedarwood, five drops of rosewood, three drops of geranium, ten drops of lavender and four drops of vetivert. Apply some oil to your hands and rub them together, warming the oil before applying it to the body.

Herbal teas

Drinking herbal teas is an excellent way of cutting down on your intake of caffeine, which causes so much stress in the West. Ginger tea puts the heat back into your digestion and can also act as a powerful anti-inflammatory. Camomile tea, which contains azulene, also has anti-inflammatory properties and may help you get to sleep at night. Coriander tea cools the body in hot weather and warms it in cool weather. Cardamom tea is excellent for dispersing phlegm or mucus from the digestive system and makes the digestion less sluggish. Stinging-nettle tea makes a fantastic diuretic. Liquorice tea is good as a liver tonic and should be taken in the morning. Fennel tea will stimulate the appetite.

Herbs and food

There are many ways in which healing herbs can be taken through your diet and only a few are suggested here. Consider using cumin as a table condiment instead of pepper for its carminative properties, expelling gas from the stomach and intestines. Cayenne pepper, called the 'king of heat' in the *Gyud Zhi*, can also be used as a condiment and benefits those at risk from heart disease. Cinnamon helps regulate blood sugar and can be sprinkled on toast and desserts. Clove is an excellent tonic for the life channel *srog rtsa* and can be added to sweet and savoury stews. Saffron, which can be used to colour rice (as in the Spanish dish *paella*), detoxifies the biological system and is a preventative against liver and heart disease.

Foods for the *nagas*

In Tibetan Buddhism, one cause of illness is thought to be the wrath of the *nagas*, the spirit guardians of place. *Nagas* become angry if their home is disturbed and may cause illness (see page 62). If you are ill, it may be that you have inadvertently interfered with their environment.

Traditionally, white foods are used as offerings to appease the wrath of the *naga* kings and to gain wealth, fame, confidence, merit and whatever else you may wish for. You can create a plate of offerings from foods like natural yogurt, white rice, white chocolate and so on. If you want to burn incense, throw powdered spices (such as cardamom, five spice or even supermarket mixed herbs) on burning charcoal. As the spice smoke is released towards heaven, make requests for your health or your dreams to all the deities. (Don't ever place raw meat on a shrine or you will cause the deities to faint!)

White foods are offered to the nagas. *Add water to flour to achieve a paste that can be moulded in a stupa-shaped bowl.*

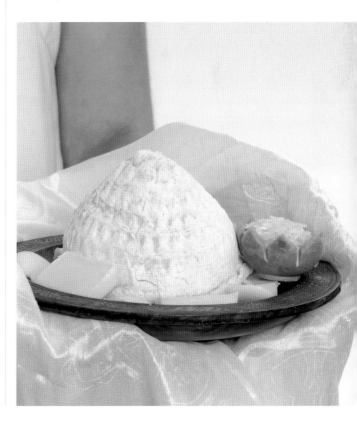

Rejuvenation programme

Tibetan medicine prescribes a rejuvenation programme (especially for those suffering stress 'burnout' and those over 60) to increase longevity and youthfulness and restore vital force to the body. The practice aims to rebalance the body's energetic systems and promote the production of the body's seven constituents: nutritional essence, blood, flesh, fat, bone, marrow and regenerative fluid. It also boosts the functioning of the excretory processes to detoxify the body. You can use this programme whenever you feel tired and in need of an energy boost.

Techniques for modern times

When the *Gyud Zhi* and *The Blue Beryl* were compiled in Tibet in the 17th century, the environment was unpolluted. Today, global industrialization has polluted everyone's land, air, water and food with heavy metals and chemicals that build up in the body, inhibiting biochemical functions and giving rise to diseases such as arthrosclerosis, cancer and Alzheimer's. The rejuvenation programme suggested here seeks to eliminate heavy metals and other pollutants from the body.

Before the retreat

Many cultures the world over teach that there is no point in putting good medicine into a dirty body. Before starting a rejuvenation programme, you must first begin to remove the accumulated toxins from the body. There are various ways in which this can be done.

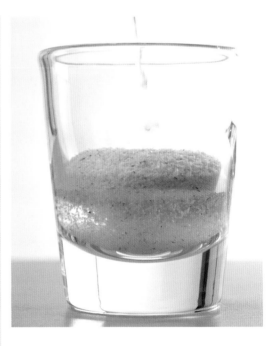

The gel formed when water is combined with psyllium husks can absorb toxins and remove them from the body.

Psyllium husks

Some Tibetan doctors recommend taking one dessertspoon of psyllium husks with half a glass of tepid water each day. When mixed with liquid, the soluble psyllium fibre forms a gel that helps remove toxins from the body. If you are planning a rejuvenation programme, try to start taking the psyllium about a week before it starts.

Purging herbs and colonic irrigation

A couple of days before starting the rejuvenation programme, you might like to take a mixture of herbs to purge your digestive system. The purging herbs must be prescribed and supplied by your doctor.

A Tibetan doctor might also recommend a pre-programme colonic irrigation with a professional therapist. Irrigating the bowels will remove the foods that may combine in a way that causes the bowel to impact and generate disease.

Milk thistle

Silybum marianum or milk thistle offers another valuable means to detoxify and rejuvenate the body before a programme begins. Milk thistle contains a compound called silymarin that protects the liver from toxins and has the ability to regenerate liver cells. Add five drops of tincture per 6.3 kg (14 lb) of your weight to a glass of warm water and drink daily three days before and three days after a juice fast.

Chelation

Some doctors of Tibetan medicine recommend a course of chelation (binding of a substance to a metal) to remove heavy metals from the body, in particular lead, cadmium and mercury. This is a simple procedure using the amino acid EDTA (ethylenediaminetetraacetic acid) administered by IV line by a conventional medical doctor at a specialist clinic. A 1989 study suggests that the therapy can also be helpful for people with coronary artery disease and other vascular problems. Chelation should usually be undergone a minimum of five days before the rejuvenation programme starts.

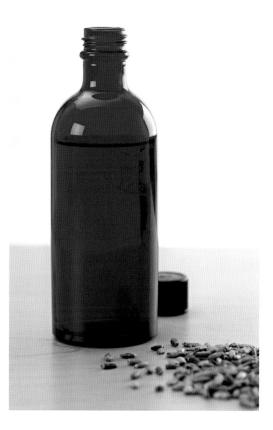

Help detoxify your body by taking tincture of milk thistle mixed with water before and after the programme.

Coriander

One simple way to chelate heavy metals out of the body naturally is to include coriander in your diet, as this herb has been scientifically proven to chelate mercury from the body. In the future, science will show what other herbs, vegetables and spices can chelate lead and cadmium, in order to maintain health and ensure the proper functioning of the body.

Following the programme

A daily programme of activities is suggested in the box. This five-day retreat includes rest, meditation and yoga, so plan to follow it when you can take time out and be free from stress. Try to retreat to a peaceful environment, ideally one surrounded by the natural world. Avoid drinking alcohol and eating eggs, fish, garlic and ginger for some days before and certainly during

Daily programme	
8.00	Breakfast
9.30	Light stretching
10–12.00	Meditation
13.00	Lunch
14.30	Yoga prostrations
16.00	Bath therapy and massage
18.00	Dinner
19.00	Chanting visualization
21.00	Retire to room

the retreat; also abstain from sexual intercourse. When not following an activity, retreatants are encouraged to take part in peaceful activities such as reading, quiet contemplation and walking in nature.

Stretching

Before your meditative practice, it is a good idea to relax your muscles with a few stretching exercises. These will release accumulated stress and prepare you for a state of serenity, helping you to gain maximum benefit from the meditative experience. Try some gentle yoga poses or the stretches shown below.

Nostril clearing

In Buddhist meditation, the mind rides the breath so it is very important to clear the body of stale airs before beginning practice. Block the right nostril with your left hand, breathe deeply into the right lung three times and exhale all the stale airs. Reverse the process to clear the left lung. This process also cleans the channels in the body especially the three main ones connected to *lung*,

tripa and *bekan* energy (see page 48). When you finish, breathe deeply in through both nostrils and you will find the influx should be balanced. Then three times inhale and exhale and when exhaling breathe out the bird of attachment, snake of anger and the pig of ignorance. You can now begin your meditation practice (see page 128 for an introduction to Buddhist meditation).

Chanting visualization

In Tantric Buddhism, a mantra is the sound of the Buddha with whom you have a karmic connection. You can chant any Buddhist mantra that you know (see pages 164–169) and as you chant try to visualize the associated deity (see page 58 for information about visualizing the Medicine Buddha). Chanting a mantra arouses a vibration that blesses and purifies your body, speech, mind and even your environment. Chanting also helps draw your attention away from discursive thinking and relaxes your nervous system in preparation for sleep. If your mind is relaxed at the end of the chanting session, meditate for ten minutes and enjoy the peace.

Stretching

It is important to breathe correctly when you are stretching. Breathe from the belly, not from your chest. Breathe in fully and exhale all the stale air.

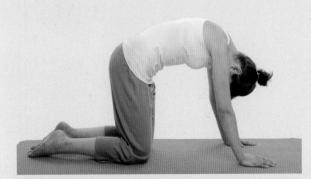

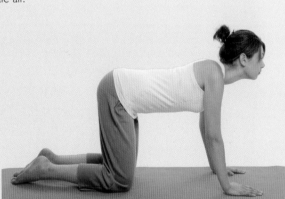

1 Kneel with hands hip-width apart. Arch up your back as high as possible, exhaling deeply. This will clear stale air from your lungs.

2 When you can't exhale any more, drop your back slowly as you draw fresh air into your body. Fill up your body completely with new air.

Bath therapy

During the programme, take a herbal bath once a day. Follow the method for making herbal baths described on page 110, using a mixture of juniper berries, lemon balm, camomile and lavender. Alternatively, ask a doctor of Tibetan medicine for a prescription for a mixture of healing herbs that will suit your constitutional type and state of health.

Aromatic oil massage

Immediately after the bath, massage your body with aromatic oil while the blood remains close to the surface of your skin, which aids absorption of the oils. To make up the aromatic oil, blend 90 ml (3¼ fl oz) sweet almond oil with 10 ml (½ fl oz) colourless sesame oil in a bottle. Sesame oil is recommended in the medical *tantras* for disorders of *lung* energy as it reduces stress. It is also thought to increase the vital essences in the body, which impart health and wellbeing and give skin a healthy glow. Add five drops of essential oils of clove, sandalwood, geranium (not to be used during pregnancy) and patchouli, then apply to the skin. Rub in the oils gently all over, stroking towards the heart to encourage lymphatic drainage and detoxification of the body. (See page 116 for more on massage.)

Rejuvenation foods

During the five-day programme, build your diet around raw vegetarian foods, in particular sprouted seeds and beans, which will provide the energy that a tired body needs. Take supplements of flaxseed oil (one tablespoon daily), which contains omega-3 essential fatty acids. Three days into the programme, introduce yogurt to replenish the bowel with probiotic bacteria and to provide B vitamins and boost immunity.

Tibetan goji berries (see page 90) are an ideal foodstuff to consume while undertaking a rejuvenation programme. Traditionally they are used for their revitalizing effect on disorders of *lung* energy, such as depression and insomnia. They are extremely high in vitamin C.

Nyung-ne fasting retreat

The tradition of *nyung-ne*, which means 'to fast and abide', was begun in the 10th century by the Princess Gelongma Palmo, after she contracted leprosy. While retreating in a forest, she had a vision of King Indrabhuti (the 8th-century King of Uddiyana), who told her to meditate on the Buddha of Compassion. In doing so, she healed her leprosy, became enlightened and began the tradition of this Tantric fasting retreat, which purifies karma, one of the causes of disease.

A full fasting retreat consists of eight two-day sessions. On the noon of the first day, a meal is eaten. On the second day there is no food or water. Six hundred prostrations (see page 138) are performed every day and the mantra of compassion is pronounced: *Om Mani Padme Hum*. This practice purifies the energy channels and patients have reported amazing emotional healing as a result. This retreat is the only time that abstinence from all food is practised in Tibetan medicine, since fasting is thought to exacerbate *lung* disorders.

Juicing

While on the programme, give your body the nutrition it needs by making your own fresh juices from organic fruit and vegetables. Aim to drink at least 600 ml (1 pint) of fresh juices a day: try beetroot, carrots, celery and tomatoes. Yellow grapefruit can detox the liver and help to re-establish the body's acid-alkaline balance. Pineapple can help thwart inflammation, as it contains bromelain, an enzyme with anti-inflammatory properties. After completing the five-day programme, you should continue to juice as part of a healthy diet.

Massage

In many ancient cultures, the power of touch was known to bring wellbeing and vitality. Many ancient healing systems incorporated massage as an essential treatment in their regimens. Scientific studies have demonstrated some of the benefits of massage, for example the stimulation of proper nerve development in infants. Touch enhances the physiological processes that are essential for life.

Ku nye

Massage therapy, known as *ku nye*, is very widely used in Tibetan medicine. To master this art can take up to three years of full-time study, including instruction from a Tibetan doctor. This unique form of treatment requires understanding of the life force or *tsog-lung* (see page 42) and the *tigle* essences (see page 58), which belongs only to practitioners of Tibetan medicine.

Treatment focuses on 15 main points on the body and seeks to unblock energy channels and increase vitality. By applying pressure to these points, a doctor of Tibetan medicine brings the three *nyepa* energies back into balance and encourages them to return to their seats within the body (see page 50). Tibetans use massage regularly to maintain their health and promote the free flow of vital energies within the body.

The massage points may be tender when touched, due to the blockage of internal energies at that point. By applying pressure to a point, the massage therapist aims to unblock it and enable the internal vital force to flow freely, thereby restoring wellbeing.

The use of oils, herbs and flour

Doctors of Tibetan medicine use oil infused with herbs and essential oils for massage. The base oil is generally sesame oil, which is believed to be excellent in the treatment of *lung* or stress. The massage oil used by Tibetan doctors is made by infusing the base oil with a synergistic formula composed of 25 or more herbs. These herbs usually include nutmeg, clove, cardamom, sandalwood, myrobalan, saffron and pomegranate. Through her website, Dr Keyzom Bhutti (see page 35) sells an excellent and effective Tibetan massage oil that has been made to a traditional formula. Alternatively, you can make your own herbal oil (see page 111).

Unique to Tibetan massage is the application of barley or chickpea flour on the body after treatment. After other forms of massage the oil on the body is either washed off or retained in place for as long as possible. Tibetan medicine, however, teaches that flour should be used to absorb the massage oil and any toxins that the oil may have drawn out from the body. Using the flour to soak up the oil from the skin can thus remove the toxins and rejuvenate the body. Other ingredients, such as powdered herbs, are sometimes added to the flour to enhance the detoxification effects.

In Tibetan medicine, massage is used primarily to combat stress. Its other main application is to treat people who have a predominantly *lung* constitution, especially when *lung* is in excess. For extreme stress, up to three massage sessions a week are recommended. Tibetan massage techniques are also a safe and effective way of achieving pain relief for women in labour.

Massage is used as a therapy in Tibetan medicine to ease stress and enable the free flowing of vital energies.

'Unique to Tibetan massage is the application of flour on the body'

Moxibustion and cupping

Moxibustion and cupping are both therapies that are similar to acupuncture in that they pay attention to the body's energy points. These techniques are used by doctors of Tibetan medicine only if changes to a patient's diet and lifestyle have failed to bring about a healing effect.

Healing with moxibustion

To perform *metsa*, or moxibustion, the doctor places a *moxa*, a small cone of woolly-textured dried herb, directly on the patient's body at the site of an energy point. He or she then lights the cone and leaves it to burn down to the skin. Cones are usually about the size of the tip of the index finger and are made of the herb mugwort (*mkhan pa*).

Moxibustion is used to treat 'cold' diseases, which arise when there are excessive amounts of *lung* and *bekan* energies in the body. The heat imparted by the burning cone to the energy point activates the energy channel to which it relates and disperses energetic blockages. The *Gyud Zhi* details 71 moxibustion points. Different points are treated, depending on the illness.

> 'The golden needle is so effective in stimulating all the energy channels that no other treatments will be required after a session'

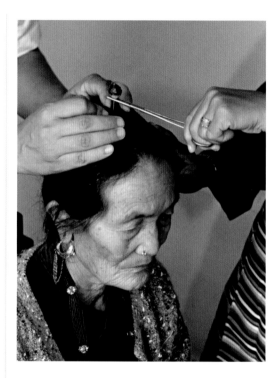

In moxibustion, herbal cones are placed on energy points on the patient's body and allowed to burn down to the skin.

The golden needle

The first method usually recommended in Tibetan medicine if moxibustion is required is the legendary golden needle technique. An acupuncture needle made from gold is inserted into the fontanelle point on the top of the head; this lies close to the crown chakra. The *moxa* is placed on top of the needle and lit and, as it burns, both the doctor and the patient chant healing mantras. As the *moxa* burns down, the airs, or vital-force winds, in the body are directed onto the correct energetic pathways. Doctors of Tibetan medicine find this technique effective for treating diseases including depression, insomnia and epilepsy, and the *Gyud Zhi* states that it can protect against nervous breakdown. Traditionally the method is also used to expel spirits and demons of possession. The golden needle technique is so effective in stimulating all the energy channels that no other treatments are required after a session.

The cupping technique

In cupping, the doctor creates a vacuum inside a number of cups using a flame, then places the cups on certain energy points on the patient's skin. The vacuum pulls the skin into an arch, which is believed to break up accumulated

Cups are used to exert suction at certain energy points in order to disperse blockages caused by built-up toxins.

toxins. The method also disperses blockages of *lung* energy. When the blood comes to the surface of the skin due to the suction, either a herbal ointment is applied to be absorbed by the blood or blood-letting takes place.

In Tibetan medicine, blood is understood to be healthy or diseased, depending on a person's lifestyle, diet, toxins, evacuations and, sometimes, spirits. Blood-letting is used to release the bad blood. A small incision is made at a blood-letting point specific to the treatment of a particular disease and a few drops of blood are released. As soon as good blood starts flowing – Tibetan doctors are able to discern the difference between good and bad blood – the letting is stopped. Blood-letting is used to treat disorders of *tripa* energy, which include blood diseases, tumours and fevers. Herbs are taken days before the treatment, causing the good and bad blood to separate in preparation for the therapy.

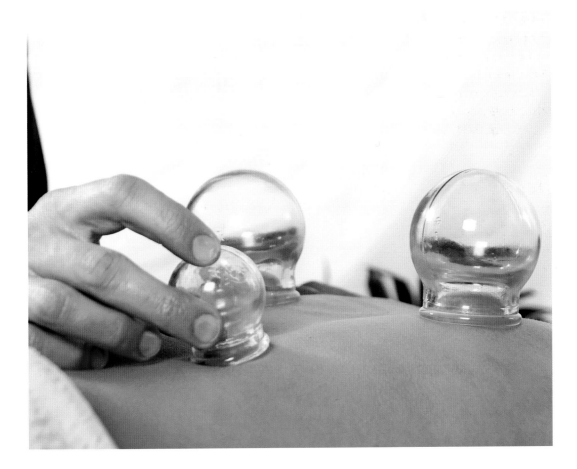

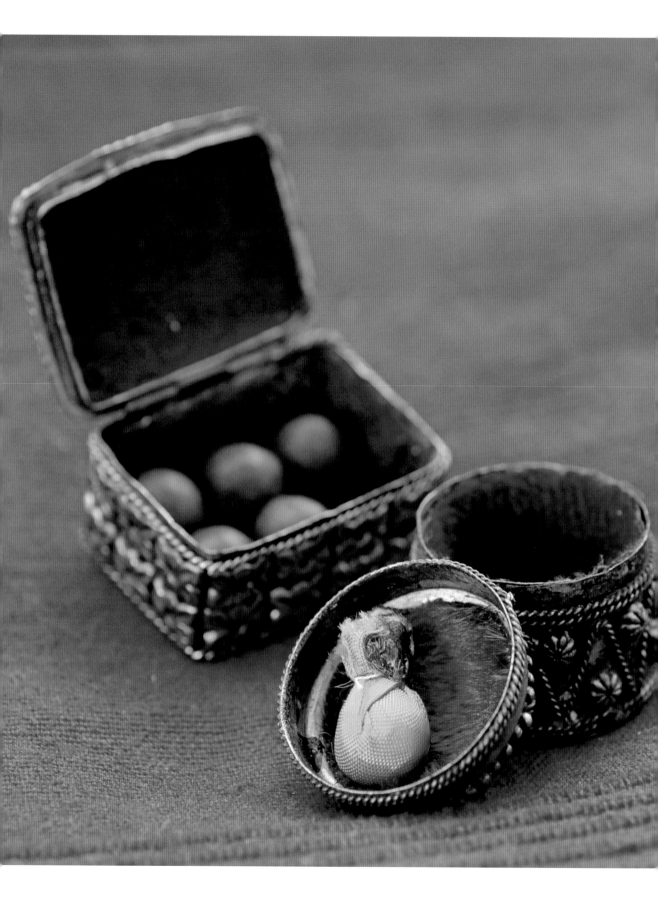

Alchemical remedies

If alchemy can be seen anywhere in the world, it's in the recipes, production and effects of the Precious Jewel Pills, unique to Tibetan medicine. The Tibetan lama doctors who create them require a profound understanding of the workings of the five elements, as well as skill as polypharmacists (pharmacists working in a number of dimensions) and medical metallurgists.

Preparation of the pills

Gold and platinum, crushed and smelted to powders, are among the ingredients used in the Tibetan alchemical remedies. Interestingly, these metals are used within Western medicine too, in the treatment of autoimmune diseases and rheumatoid arthritis, and in anti-cancer drugs.

Some of the recipes for these famed medicines date from the 13th century. One pill may contain more than 100 ingredients and take up to 40 days to produce, using a complicated pharmaceutical process and secret Tantric ritual. The pills must never see the light of day, so manufacture is carried out by candlelight and the pills are stored in candlelight, too. They are supplied wrapped in a protective cloth.

Part of the *Kalachakra Tantra*, the Tantric calendar (see page 76), is used to prepare the Precious Jewel Pills because it outlines a way of purifying and detoxifying mercury. Mercury is mechanically cleansed, heated for days and then mixed with sulphur to create mercuric sulphide, or cinnabar (this is not the same as a toxic heavy metal because it has been changed chemically and alchemically). Gold, silver, copper, different types of iron and eight minerals are added, and these substances, along with the mercury, are detoxified and alchemically transformed from a shiny liquid to a matt-black inert substance called

Precious Jewel Pills like this Dalai Lama Jewel Pill must be stored in a protective wrapping.

Taking the pills

They must be taken at astrologically favourable times, such as the dawn of a full-moon day (other auspicious days can be established from Tibetan calendars that are widely available online). Just before going to bed, dim the lights and unwrap the pill. Gently crush it in a cup, add some boiled water and cover with a clean cloth. Then go to sleep. At dawn, stir the mixture with your index finger in a clockwise direction while reciting the Medicine Buddha mantra (see page 167), then drink the solution. Return to bed and recite the Medicine Buddha mantra again, 108 times or until you fall asleep. You may find that you start to sweat; this is your body ridding itself of toxins.

You should try to avoid the following for at least two days before taking the pill and at least two days afterwards: meat and eggs; raw vegetables and fruit; uncooked grains; garlic and onion; sour, spicy or salty foods; alcoholic drinks; rancid food. Also avoid strenuous physical activities, sexual intercourse and cold baths. Traditionally, alchemical cures were often taken following a blood-letting process (see page 119).

bhasma, which is believed to be the king of antidotes to poisoning and pollution. These powders, made from precious metals through religious rites, are sacred substances, the healing ambrosia nectar of the Medicine Buddha.

Precious Jewel Pills should be taken under the supervision of a doctor of Tibetan medicine. Alternatively, they can be worn as an amulet against disease. They are available online for purchasing, for example through the website of the Mentseekhang in Dharamsala. A few of the different Precious Jewel Pills created by Tibetan lamas are described below.

The Karmapa Black Pill Rinchen Rilnack

This miracle pill is manufactured from gemstones, metals, animal and plant products by the Karmapa (the head of the Kagyu lineage of Tibetan Buddhism) in a secret ceremony with his closest disciples, using the relics of the 11th-century luminaries of Tibetan Buddhism, Marpa the Translator and Milarepa, who founded the Kagyu lineage. In a miraculous production process, 'mother' pills are placed in the begging bowel of the 3rd Karmapa (1296–1376) and the bowl is then covered with his robe overnight. Next morning the pills have multiplied, and the 'baby' pills are believed to have a multiplying capacity, too. The pills are used to alleviate depression and eradicate trauma, help a dying person connect with the Karmapa and bring about remission from disease.

Precious Wish-Fulfilling Jewel

This pill contains 16 valuable metals, plus 70 other ingredients, including purified gold, silver, copper and iron; gems such as coral, turquoise, pearl, lapis lazuli, and the rare indigenous gem of Tibet, the *zhi* stone. Cloves, bamboo and nutmeg are included, among other plant substances. The pill is renowned as an antidote to all kinds of poisoning and is useful in relieving the harmful effects of over-exposure to the sun. Tibetan doctors also prescribe it to treat paralysis and limb problems, nerve disorders and conditions of sensory impairment, such as deafness and the loss of smell, and for heart conditions and blood clots, ulcers and cancer. A healthy person can take this pill as a general tonic.

Great Cold Compound Precious Black Pill

This pill contains more than 100 ingredients, including gold, silver, copper and iron, as well as detoxified forms of the precious stones sapphire, emerald, turquoise, ruby and diamond, and a large amount of herbs. It is used especially for diseases connected with modern environmental pollution, such as radioactive heavy metals, and traditionally offers protection from contagious diseases and evil spirits.

Precious Coral 25 Rinchen Jumar

First formulated by the ancient physician Shasandhara Lakhsmi, who used the medicine to save his life, this pill is made from 25 ingredients, including detoxified coral, pearl and lapis lazuli, saffron, nutmeg and myrobalan or arura – the tree of health (see page 106). This pill is recommended for severe headaches, brain and memory disorders, fainting spells and seizures, and disorders of the nervous system. The cool nature of the coral combats fevers caused by toxins, neuritis and chronic ailments. Healthy people take this pill as a preventive measure against nerve disorders.

Elixir pills

Tibetan yogis on long meditative retreats in the mountains reciting mantras are reputed to be able to live solely on specially made herbal pills for days, weeks and, in some cases, months. These elixirs, called *chulen*, made from what are known as the five essences and four nectars (yogurt, milk, butter, honey and sugar) have come to be known in English as 'essence extraction pills'. Each one is about the size of a marble and can be taken following a detox.

Ordinary herbal pills are dried by the sun, unlike the Jewel Pills which must not be exposed to light during production.

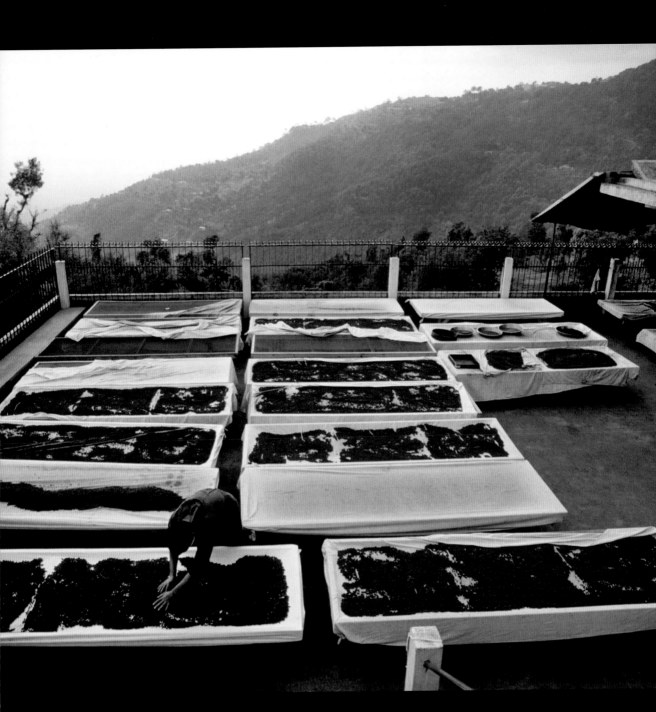

'One pill may contain more than
100 ingredients and take up to
40 days to produce'

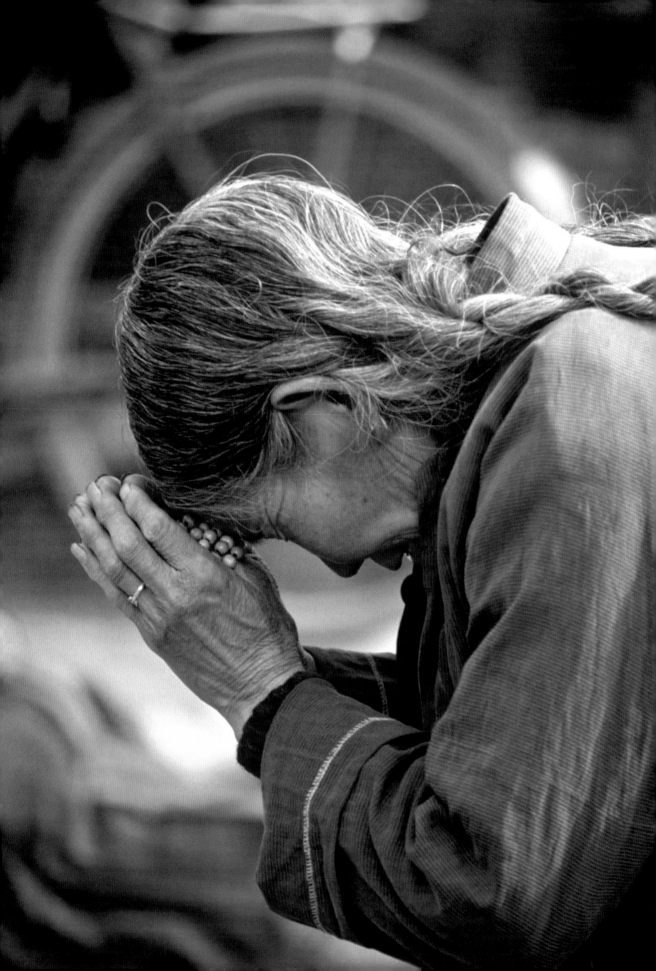

Inner space

In Tibet a healthy body with balanced life forces is
considered essential for Tantric spiritual practice.
Indeed, the fundamental aim of Tibet's ancient, unique
and complete medical system is not just mental and
physical harmony, but the spiritual enlightenment of
both patient and practitioner. Daily meditation is the
practice recommended to bring about inner and outer
balance and ultimately to lead to enlightenment. This
chapter also examines more esoteric Tantric religious
practices and Buddhist ways of thinking, which may
be helpful in the West in the treatment of ailments
of the nervous and endocrine systems and reduce the
need for conventional medication. Understanding
this integrative approach to medicine can only make
modern Western medicine more effective.

Exploring the spiritual life

If IQ assesses the 'what, where and when' of life, and emotional intelligence (or EQ) looks at the 'how', then spiritual intelligence (or SQ) is the 'why' that directs your IQ and EQ, to give life meaning. Tibetan medicine urges practitioners and patients alike to explore their spiritual lives, and ultimately insists that only by doing so can we find health and wellbeing.

A true spiritual path

Buddhists regard three terms as an unsurpassable description of the spiritual path: view, meditation and compassionate action. View refers to finding a psycho-spiritual openness as vast as space – the mind's true nature. Meditation relates to the cultivation of *bodhicitta,* an enlightened heart (see page 154), through the union of emptiness and skilful means. Action becomes spontaneously compassionate when view and meditation are realized through training by a master and diligent practice. If view and meditation are correct, actions simply improve, benefiting others. If, after exploring view and meditation, behaviour does not improve, the first two concepts have not been understood or integrated.

For example, a mental notion of what meditation is can never be enough: meditation must be experienced through practice. During meditation, it is crucial to reconnect with the body and the subtle energetics, but many people use thinking to dissociate themselves from this. Action can be provocative, too, testing the extent to which we have surpassed an egoic view of the world and arrived into freedom and spacious awareness.

In this way, the sincere practice of Tibetan Buddhism helps us to reconnect to what is real, meaningful and lasting – loving and being loved. Ultimately it leads us to find the Buddha in our hearts, a discovery that can eradicate aeons of suffering, karma, loneliness and delusion.

The health benefits of a spiritual life

In 1997 V.S. Ramachandran informed the world of neuroscience that there is a neural basis for religious experience. Scientists have shown that the feeling of oneness associated with an experience of sacredness comes about when the temporal lobe of the brain is activated by neural oscillations, or brainwaves, of 40 cycles per second (Hz). People who live spiritual, contemplative lives often activate this area of the brain and neurotheologists have come to refer to it as the 'god spot'.

Spiritual materialism

Through the ages the spiritual path of mystical traditions has concerned the destruction of the ego, or selfish world view. However, today this

---

Finding your path

Be careful where you take refuge from the materialistic world. The Tibetan Buddhist teacher Patrul Rinpoche (1808–1887) said, 'The student who doesn't examine the teacher may as well go and drink poison. The teacher who doesn't examine the student may as well go and leap off a cliff.' True meditation masters in the Tibetan Tantric tradition may take up to three years to accept a student.

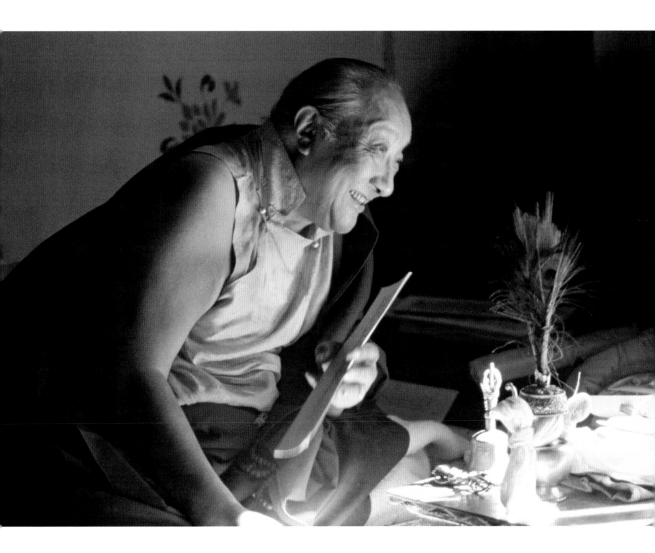

Dzogchen teacher to the Dalai Lama, Dilgo Khyentse Rinpoche (1910–1991) was one of the world's great lamas.

method is often hijacked by those in search of egoic bliss. In *Cutting Through Spiritual Materialism*, meditation master Chogyam Trungpa Rinpoche (1939–1987) urged the importance of moving away from 'spiritual materialism':

> 'It is important to see that the main point of any spiritual practice is to step out of the bureaucracy of ego. This means stepping out of ego's constant desire for a higher, more spiritual, more transcendental version of knowledge, religion, virtue, judgement, comfort or whatever it is that a particular ego is seeking. One must step out of spiritual materialism.'

Spiritual materialism is the ego's desire for more and more spiritual learning. Egoic mentality can mean simply swapping a worldly persona for a religious one. The spiritual supermarket is now so large that the egoic intellect may binge on so much knowledge and philosophy. Instead of becoming more selfless through practice, there is a danger that we can evolve into heartless *dharma* intellectuals. This is particularly relevant in the case of Tibetan Buddhism, which is vast and profound and requires an authentic guide. Those who believe that they are on a spiritual path, but who are in fact practising spiritual materialism and hanging on to ego, are likely to suffer problems with their nervous system and mental illness.

Meditation in Tibetan medicine

The health of the human spirit is a cornerstone of Tibetan medicine and the main form of practice that ensures this inner health is meditation. In the Tibetan tradition, the practice of meditation begins with understanding the thought process and gradually becomes more sophisticated. Tibetan Buddhism offers a path for this process. These techniques have been adopted by millions of people in the West for their proven stress-reducing effects. Meditation has become the holistically minded Westerner's spiritual treasure.

The meditation path

There are two aspects to meditation training in Tibetan Buddhism, *shamatha* and *vispassana*. In *shamatha*, the meditator focuses the mind by turning his or her attention to the breath, a technique that calms the thinking mind. The calming process has several stages: traditionally

Formal sitting meditation is a central practice for the monks of Tibet's Buddhist monasteries.

the mind is pictured first as a waterfall, then as a fast-flowing river, later as a calm river and finally as the point at which the river meets the ocean. The progression from stage to stage depends on the individual.

Vispassana is analytical meditation. Its practice is an experiential process of dismantling the egoic self. You are ready to start *vispassana* meditation once you have done some *shamatha* meditation and feel that you can graduate to this

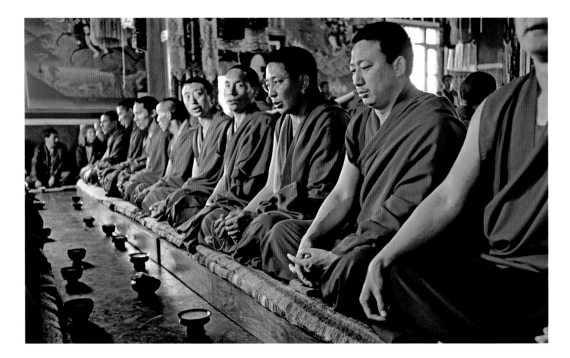

method. The practice of *Vispassana* meditation arrests the intellect and gradually releases or unveils the true mind, permitting a detached, luminous, crisp, alert and pristine awareness. In this way *vispassana* meditation allows those who practise to put the ego-centred self on hold. The Buddha once said, 'If you see the trap, you don't get caught.'

Those who practise meditation can begin the journey home to the heart. Meditation brings about relaxation and thus release from the stress of modern living, but it is much more than this. It is a profound spiritual journey and it is best to work with a master to achieve results. Studying with a master for one day is said to be more effective than 1,000 days of reading, since to voyage into the mind you require a guide who knows the way.

The aim of meditation

In Tibetan Buddhism, meditation is a path towards understanding *shunyata*, the Buddhist principle of emptiness or openness. Put simply, *shunyata* defines the truth that there is no 'self'. This is the only reality. The Mahasiddha Aryadeva (3rd century CE) said that even to consider whether or not all things are empty in nature causes duality (and more importantly *samsara*, or egoic consciousness) to fall asunder.

The Buddhist understanding of self

Tibetan Buddhism teaches that every person is born innocent. As young children, we are often allowed, depending on our family circumstances, to be free-spirited and to express this original love. Then comes the time when we arrive at school and our natural view begins to be controlled. Our sense of wonder becomes buried beneath a pile of intellectual information. The way in which we relate to the world shifts from the heart to the brain, as our sense of self becomes more profound and our separation from others widens. The Buddha teaches that this sense of an apparently solid self is the underlying cause of all our woes.

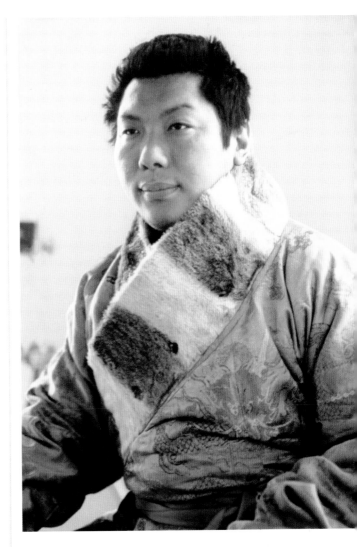

An enlightened master, such as the founder of Shambhala, Chogyam Trungpa Rinpoche (1939–1987), may be said to exist in a permanent meditative state of mahamudra.

We hone this sense of self as we grow up, and it comes to define our confidence, self-esteem and mental wellbeing. But all these qualities rest on thin ice because they are based on a creation – who we are, the self – that simply doesn't exist. Perpetual fear and anxiety result because the edifice can collapse at any time (and invariably it does), since all phenomena are impermanent. The only genuine, lasting and reliable self-confidence and psychological security comes from discovering the sky-like and stainless nature of our true mind, the original innocence with which we were born – our Buddha nature. We achieve this through the practice of meditation.

The health benefits of meditation

Life in the West leads us to experience a great deal of stress. Tibetan Buddhism understands that it is our education and thinking that are the ultimate cause of our anxieties, because they lead us to believe that what we need lies outside us, in the form of possessions. Such expectations set us up for a life of competitiveness and selfishness, which makes us sick and distracts us from the genuine wellbeing that we truly need.

True wellbeing comes from love, a feeling of belonging and community, satisfaction with what we have, realistic expectations and a sane partner. Tibetan medicine teaches us how to use meditation to step off the materialistic treadmill.

Studies suggest that, in addition to offering relaxation, meditation boosts the effectiveness of the immune system and even 'rewires' the brain. For example, a study of American health-insurance statistics carried out on more than 2,000 people practising meditation over a five-year period found that meditators consistently experienced less than half the hospitalization of other comparable groups and fewer incidents of illness in 17 medical treatment categories, including heart disease and cancer. Those who meditated were found to visit their doctor 50 per cent less than other groups. Other studies have shown that meditation can control high blood pressure as effectively as medication, and can also alleviate symptoms of PMT.

In 1997, a radiologist at the University of Pennsylvania discovered why meditation can boost immunity and ease mental stress. He showed that during meditation the brain does not shut down, but shifts its energy and blood to different parts of the brain, especially those connected with immunity and the emotions. In studies of what has come to be called the 'relaxation response', Herbert Benson, a Harvard researcher, has shown that those who practise transcendental meditation use less oxygen during meditation and that their heart rate is lowered and their pre-sleep brainwaves are increased.

Practical meditation

In *The Dalai Lama's Secret Temple*, Ian Baker quotes Garab Dorje, the first human master of the Tibetan Dzogchen teachings, on the practice of meditation:

> *'Mind's nature is Buddha from the beginning.*
> *It has neither birth nor cessation, like space.*
> *When you realize the real meaning of the equal*
>   *nature of all things*
> *To remain in that state without searching*
>   *is meditation.'*

Beginning the practice of meditation is the greatest thing you can do to benefit your life and that of those around you. For many thousands of years, meditation has been practised according to different traditions. In Buddhism, meditation is not practised just for relaxation, but as a method to attain enlightenment itself. Therefore both the practice of meditation and the cross-legged posture that is commonly depicted of Buddhas are intensely sacred.

All suffering comes from the mind; ultimate freedom comes from a study of the mind. Meditation aims to reduce mental activity and begin the process of deconstruction of egocentricity or self-centredness. The goal of meditation is to make you aware of your inner space and how vast it is. Meditation is the laboratory in which you deconstruct the self. When the mind starts to look inward, rather than reacting to everything outside, this it is said to be the beginning of *nirvana*.

When you start meditation, do small sessions of five to ten or 15 minutes. Build up the habit of practising through short daily sessions, moving on to more extended periods. An excellent time to practise meditation is in the morning, when you wake up. It shouldn't be hard to build a short session into your routine at this hour and it will set you up for the rest of the day. Begin with

The seven physical postures

As we have seen, the methods commonly employed in Tantric Buddhism are *shamatha* and *vispassana* – the former meaning 'calm abiding' and the latter 'clear insight'. *Shamatha* needs to be mastered first. As you begin its practice, you should employ seven physical postures that all the enlightened masters have used. These seven postures form the basis of Buddhist meditation and stimulate mental clarity.

7 Keeping the mind relaxed

When the mind is relaxed, its true nature begins to dawn. At first your awareness will detach itself from your thinking and start witnessing your state of thinking. Traditionally your meditation journey is described in the following stages: a waterfall, rapids, fast-moving water, calm water and finally merging with the ocean.

4 Keeping the eyes open

The eyes must be open. As you start meditation, you can close them for a little while to calm down the mind. The Buddha turned the wheel of the *Dharma* three times: the first time he said there was mind; the second time he said there was no mind; and the third time he said mind was luminous. If you don't meditate with the eyes open, you may not come to understand the nature of your mind or its luminosity. Start your practice with your gaze downwards at 45 degrees to calm the mind. If you get sleepy, raise your gaze upwards for a little while, then go back to gazing at 45 degrees.

6 Keeping the shoulders straight and the chin tucked in

By keeping the shoulders straight and relaxed you will be less tense. This also forces the chest out, giving you a sense of divine pride and open-heartedness that is characteristic of a *bodhisattva* warrior. When the chin is out, the mind is oriented to the future and its numerous possibilities.

5 Putting the tongue against the palate

The tip of the tongue placed against the palate is believed to connect all the internal energies in a way that enables the subtle life energies to flow. You will not have to swallow as much, for the saliva will simply flow down your throat and not interrupt your meditation. Experienced practitioners can meditate for periods of up to three hours and beyond.

3 Keeping the spine straight

The spine must be kept straight as a stack of golden coins; there must be no slouching. Osteopaths and chiropractors are well aware how lack of proper posture impacts on your health, including interference with nerve signals. In Tibetan medicine, the *rtsa* or channels must not be constricted, so that energy may flow correctly through the body.

1 Sitting with the legs in the *vajra* position

This is the crossed-leg posture. Placing the legs in this position encourages the internal energies of the body to become balanced and helps you to remain alert. If you try to practise meditation while walking around, your mind will be busy; if you try it lying down, you could drift off and lose your focus.

2 Placing the hands in the meditation *mudra*

In Tantric Buddhism there are many beautiful *mudras* or hand gestures, each with its own meaning (see page 132). For the purpose of meditation, the *dhyana mudra* is usually used. In this *mudra*, the left hand is placed palm up, and the right hand is placed palm up on top, with the thumbs just touching. When we are in mental activity we use our hands to express what we mean and by the position of the hands we can also help the mind come to rest.

Mudras of the Medicine Buddha

The eight *mudras* shown below are *mudras* of offering to the Medicine Buddha and
his *devas* (angels) and can be performed daily as part of meditation practice.

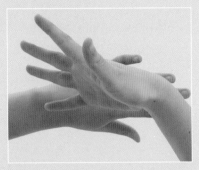

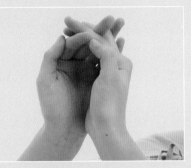

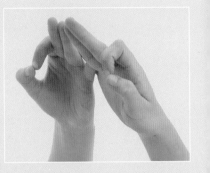

1 Prepare yourself to begin the
sequence of Medicine Buddha
mudras by rolling your hands one over
the other.

2 **Argham mudra** Representing a
pitcher, this *mudra* signifies the
offering of drinking water.

3 **Padyam mudra** Representing a basin,
this *mudra* signifies the offering of
water for washing the feet.

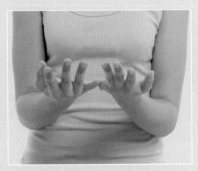

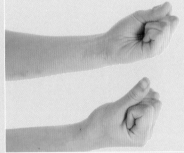

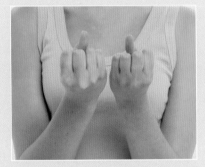

4 **Pushpe mudra** This *mudra* illustrates
the offering of flowers to the
Medicine Buddha.

5 **Dhupe mudra** Representing sticks
of incense, this *mudra* signifies the
offering of incense.

6 **Aloke mudra** Representing two
flickering flames, this *mudra* signifies
the offering of light.

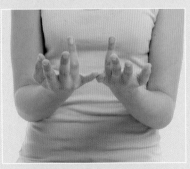

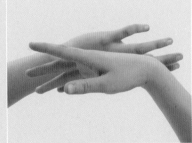

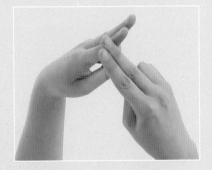

7 **Gandhe mudra** Representing the
parting of a cloth, this *mudra*
signifies the offering of perfume.

8 **Naivadya mudra** This *mudra*
illustrates the offering of food.

9 **Shapta mudra** Representing
clashing cymbals, this *mudra*
signifies the offering of music.

breath-watching *shamatha* meditation, then move on to *vispassana* when you are ready.

At no time should you be forceful in your practice, as this can cause the *lung* energy to become aggravated. Some days your practice will go well and other days maybe not, but never give up. Keep going because what you are bringing forth could be of great benefit to humankind. The realignment of energy forces in the body caused by meditation is more of a process than an event. This process needs time and the more it is enjoyed, the better the result.

Study the Seven Points of Mind Training, a tradition developed to stop you falling back into mental delusion. These seven points are divided into a total of 52 easy-to-remember slogans, such as: 'Don't expect applause', 'Don't bring things to a painful point', 'In post-meditation be a child of illusion'. These help tame the mind, increase awareness and enhance your meditation. They can also protect the mind from being flooded by ego games, which may try to keep you living in the darkness of *marigpa*, or the delusory self.

The *mudras*

In Tantric Buddhism, *mudras* are the symbolic gestures, made using the hands and fingers, which are employed in rituals. They reflect an enlightened state and are often depicted being used by Buddhas and deities in Tantric paintings. *Mudras* personify different powers embodied by the Buddha or deity and they each have a different meaning. The standard *mudra* used in meditation is the *dhyana mudra* (see page 131), but you can make others part of your daily ritual.

'When there are lots of thoughts, follow the breath' From the Buddha's *Dhammapada*

Sky Treasury *mudra*

This practice was taught to Prince Mutisenpo, son of King Tritsong Detsen, by Padmasambhava so that he could practise to become enlightened.

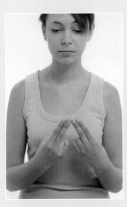 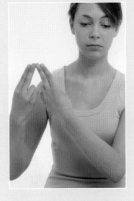 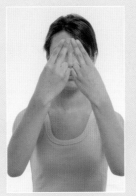 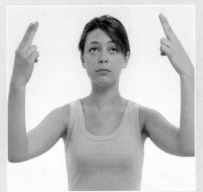

1 Bring your two forefingers together to symbolize the merging of male and female energies.

2 Holding the finger position, move the *mudra* in a circular direction clockwise and upwards.

3 At this point, the *mudra* symbolizes the moment of enlightenment.

4 As you open your arms, the *mudra* symbolizes the sky and the enlightened spacious mind of total awareness.

The brain versus the heart

If you ask Tibetans where the mind is, they gesture to the heart. They may even find the question strange – the answer is so obvious to them. To the average Westerner, the mind is in the brain. In fact, our whole cultural self-understanding is connected to the brain, which may help account for the tensions experienced within a modern lifestyle. Tibetan Buddhism and its system of medicine show us a way to return to a more health-giving, heart-focused way of life.

Restoring peace in the brain

Western science has explained how the amygdala is the part of our brain connected to emotional states. It comprises two nerve groups the size of almonds that activate the sympathetic nervous system. This system manages stress through a biochemical fight-or-flight response. At the first perception of danger, it switches to red alert: the heart rate increases, the mouth dries and blood flows away from the digestive system to prepare the muscles for action. The neurons in the amygdala react so quickly that the physical response outperforms any thinking action. Emotional experiences, especially negative ones, imprinted in the synapses in the amygdala trigger this stress response. Even a minor stimulus that resembles a previous negative experience, such as a facial expression or a ringing phone, can trigger that same biochemical reaction.

When this reaction continues for some time and is often repeated, it can contribute to chronic health conditions, ranging from heart disease to depression. In the West we tend to live in a state of constantly triggered stress response – in traffic jams, with work deadlines – which makes it essential that we learn how to turn on the parasympathetic nervous system that reverses the body's stress symptoms. Meditation does this so effectively because it causes the body to shift from a state of red alert to one of relaxation.

Release of the 'love hormone', oxytocin, subdues the amygdala and its fear responses. Sincere practice and study of Tibetan Buddhism and meditation will stimulate the release of oxytocin and so return the mind to peace.

Buddhism and the brain

Tibetan Buddhism regards the brain as just another sense organ, and thinking as a means of reinforcing the delusory sense of self that causes all our suffering. We may spend years sharpening a highly prized intellect, but this structure is mere delusion and gives rise to disorders of *lung* energy. If our thinking suddenly comes to a halt, rather than embracing openness we are terrified (since we understand who we are as 'thinking') and recoil into our deluded state of 'why-because' thinking and material ambition. In order to return to an innate state of harmony and health, we need to disengage the brain and relate to our lives and the world from the heart.

Returning to the heart

In all forms of medicine in Asia, the heart is referred to as an emperor. In Tibetan medicine, the life-force channel (*srog rtsa*) is situated near the heart. When the channel is disturbed by an

Avalokiteshvara, the Bodhisattva of Compassion, symbolizes the heart-centred nature of Tibetan Buddhism.

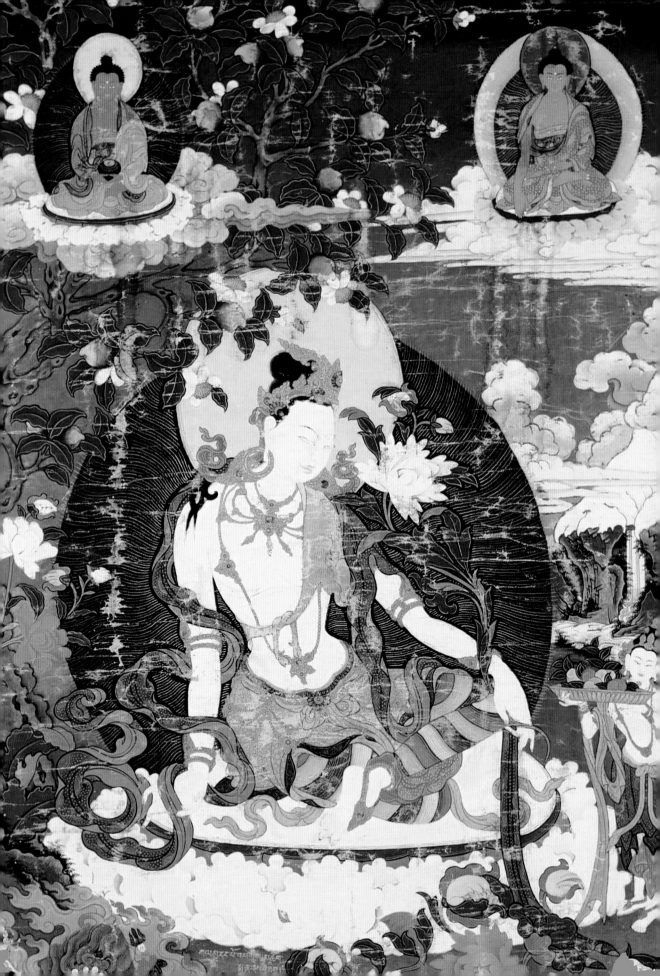

imbalance in *lung* energy, mental illness ensues. Tantric healers also teach that those searching for material power often suffer from heart disease. Meditation and other healing techniques seek to harmonize the three life energies. The heart channel can be calmed by an easy-to-use technique known as heart coherence (see box).

Mind-body medicine

In Western society we tend to dissociate our minds from our bodies. We become human 'doings' rather than human 'beings', consumers rather than citizens, and so create a values vacuum that is destroying our planet through our dissociation from nature and the five elements.

The heart may be the healing link that helps us re-establish a connection between the mind and the body. According to Tibetan mystical anatomy, at the centre of the heart resides a sphere of *bodhi* or enlightened mind substance. This heart drop, or luminous Buddha sphere in the heart, is the source of all the *tigles* that pervade the body (see page 58). By encouraging love, we restore balance to this fundamental system of human health – and the wider world.

Recent scientific research by Dr Candace Pert, who has discovered a communication network in the body running through the immune system, seems to confirm the heart-mind link. She describes a bodywide memory system made up of neuropeptides and their receptors, supported by the heart and the thymus gland. These neuropeptides pervade the body in what Pert describes as a 'psychoimmunoendocrine' system (relating to body, mind and spirit). Understanding these ideas can bring about a paradigm shift in how we protect our health – by loving.

This Tibetan medical illustration depicts the energy channels found at the heart.

Performing heart coherence

Begin by sitting and, as you inhale, visualize breathing into the heart area (not the heart organ, but the heart of yourself) and focus your attention there. Try doing this as you hold a crystal to your heart chakra. Imagine a feeling of love, and let it trigger warmth and peace in your chest area. This tells the emotional brain that everything is okay, and thus the nervous system becomes balanced. Relax as you inhale and exhale, for about 20 minutes. If your heart is still not coherent, watch it become so as you continue breathing. Do this technique daily until you get the hang of relaxing physically while remaining mentally alert.

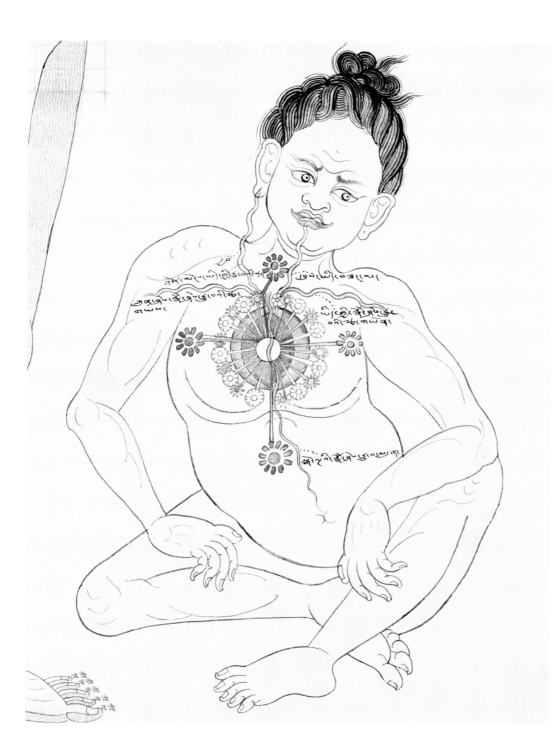

'The intuitive mind is a sacred gift and
the rational mind a faithful servant'

Albert Einstein

Yoga in Tibetan medicine

A spiritual system that was practised at least 2,000 years ago, yoga seeks to unite the mind, spirit and body as one. Its eight-branched system leads students through practices that cleanse mind and body, control the breath and foster meditation, devotion and selfless service, to bring about liberation and absolute bliss.

One of the branches of yoga, asana, or physical movements, has become popular in the West since the 1960s as a means of keeping fit and releasing tension. It is accepted that exercise is essential for good health and yoga is an ideal form of exercise. For example, the postures of physical yoga give every part of the body a massage and they also remove stale waste-bearing

Doing a yoga prostration

As you do the prostrations, repeat the Prayer to the Three Jewels: 'I take refuge in the Buddha. I take refuge in the *Dharma*. I take refuge in the *Sangha*.'

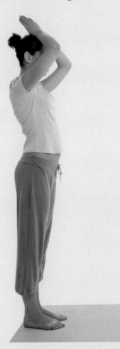

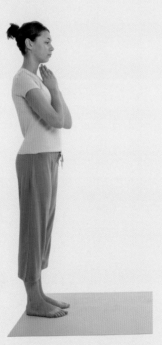

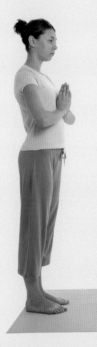

1 To begin the prostration, place your hands on your head to symbolize purification of body.

2 Place your hands against your throat to symbolize purification of speech.

3 Place your hands against your heart to symbolize purification of mind.

fluids such as lymph, allowing new nutrient-rich fluids to access the cells. All forms of exercise promote flow of lymph, but yoga in particular helps its replenishment. Breathing is taught in most systems of yoga, and breathing deeply – for some people, breathing properly for the first time – sends more oxygen to the cells and expels carbon dioxide. Yoga postures also massage the internal organs and tone the digestive system, enhancing its function. The immediate effect of practising yoga is stimulation of the 'relaxation response' (see page 130).

The practice of yoga has been shown to stimulate sensory receptors all over the body, keeping the body healthy and helping us make sense of the world. For example, impulses from nerve endings relay information from the sense organs to the brain, where it is processed and stimulates impulses to move muscles and activate the endocrine glands. Without these impulses the body degenerates. Doctors of Tibetan medicine particularly recommend yoga for those with arthritis and those suffering from low vitality.

However, yoga is not just practised to stay fit. By balancing the energies in the body, yoga makes meditation effective. Performing a prostration (shown below) purifies karma and rids us of negative emotions and consequently of disease. The ultimate aim of yoga is to enable spiritual evolution towards enlightenment.

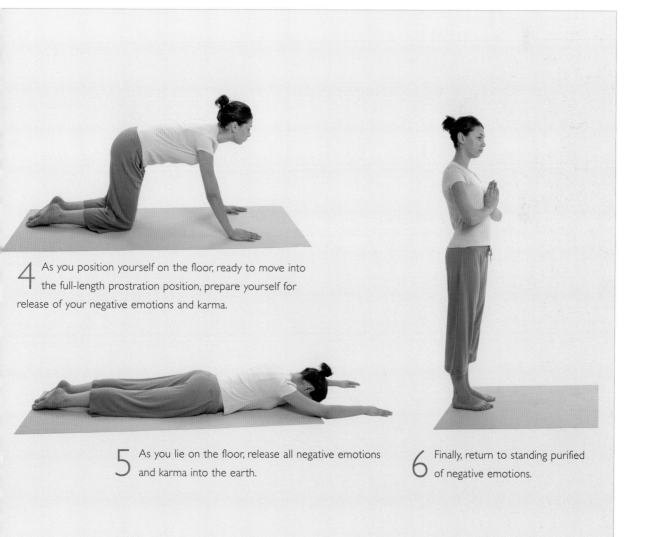

4 As you position yourself on the floor, ready to move into the full-length prostration position, prepare yourself for release of your negative emotions and karma.

5 As you lie on the floor, release all negative emotions and karma into the earth.

6 Finally, return to standing purified of negative emotions.

Tibetan exercise

In *The Ancient Secret of the Fountain of Youth*, Peter Kelder described the physical postures of the Five Rites: spinning with the arms extended; lying on the floor with the legs in the air; kneeling and arching backwards; feet and hands on the floor pushing the stomach upwards; and a cobra-like pose. The authenticity of the exercises has never been confirmed or denied, but the postures are believed to slow down the ageing process and increase energy levels, and it only takes ten minutes to do the 21 repetitions of each movement. More than two million copies of Kelder's book have been sold.

Yantra yoga

In fact, a system of Tibetan yoga, called yantra yoga or *trul khor*, evolved many centuries ago as a method to open the subtle-body mandalas (internal energy centres), but until recently was shrouded in secrecy. The system comprises 108 movements performed not as static poses but as a continuous sequence, somewhat faster than a t'ai chi class, together with breath control. To complete the movements takes up to ten hours, but Lama Lobsang, who lives in Chicago, has designed a 90-minute class based on the system.

Originally taught in the 8th century by Vairochana (see page 30), a student of Padmasambhava who had learnt them from the Nepalese Mahasiddha Humkara, the movements of yantra yoga have been passed down through the ages in an unbroken secret lineage. In order to preserve them as a living tradition, certain lineage holders have now released some of the movements to the world. To help conserve the tradition for the future practitioners of Tantric Buddhism, parts of some of the movements are depicted on the next three pages. However, they are not intended for the uninitiated to practise at home. To master yantra yoga requires instruction from a guru who holds the secret lineage.

Breathing plays such an important role in *trul khor* because it affects the body's life force. These three aspects (posture, movement and holding the breath), when implemented simultaneously, create an effect that rejuvenates the psychic energies in the body and the channels that contain them. The physical movements, too, bring the body's three vital energies into balance, which is considered the essence of health in Tibetan medicine. Practising these movements removes blocks in the *rtsa* energy channels (see page 48), allowing consciousness to pervade the body. This results in the practice of clear light where no 'I' exists: all the life energies in the body are in balance, the mind becomes extremely clear, and you see the luminosity of your mind and become stable in it.

During the movements, the attention of the mind is focused on the chakras (see page 56), causing them to be more vibrant. By harmonizing the *rtsa channels*, *lung* and *tigle* drops and balancing the five elements internally, a practitioner brings the sun and moon energies of the psychic body to union at the navel. Here, at the base of the central energy channel, is the location for the mystic heat called *tummo*, which, when produced by yogis, brings about internal bliss (see page 144).

'In yantra yoga the asana, or position, is one of the important points but not the main one. Movement is more important'

Namkhai Norbu, *Yantra Yoga*

Movements of yantra yoga

These secret and sacred movements are illustrated here for reference purposes only. Do not attempt them without guidance from a qualified master.

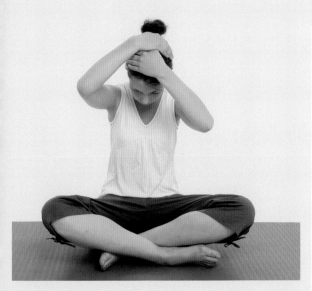

Opening the crown chakra

One hand is moved over the other across the head in order to stimulate the gallbladder meridian and the crown chakra.

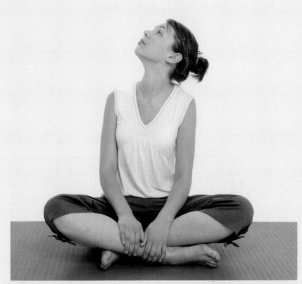

Lion's breath

Air is inhaled sharply through the nose on one side of the body and then the other in order to clear the practitioner's channels of stale air.

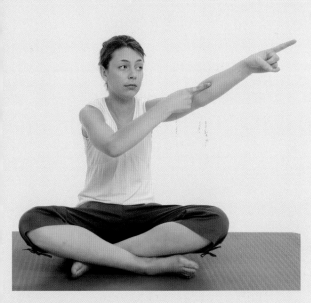

Pulling the bow

The fingertip is drawn down the arm as if drawing back a bow string, to open the heart meridian and the chest.

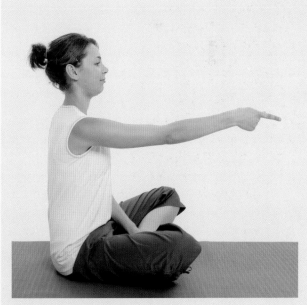

Firing the finger

The fingers are thrown outwards, to cause the internal psychic system to align itself correctly.

Movements of yantra yoga

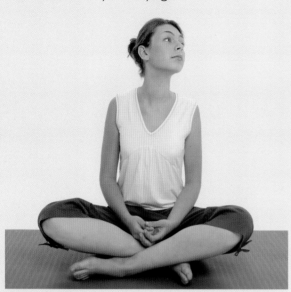

Opening the throat chakra

The practitioner rolls the head in a clockwise direction and then in an anticlockwise direction, in order to open up the throat chakra.

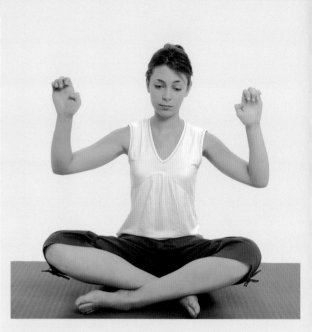

Hooking the air

The arms are raised to head height, with palms open and fingers bent over. The hands are then drawn down in a hooking position at the same time as the practitioner breathes out, exhaling stale air from the body.

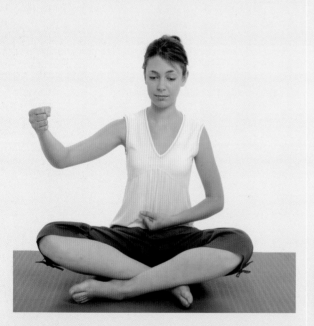

Activating the navel

This movement, in which the belly is repeatedly pounded, is performed by yogis and yoginis to activate the mystic fire, *tummo*, at the navel.

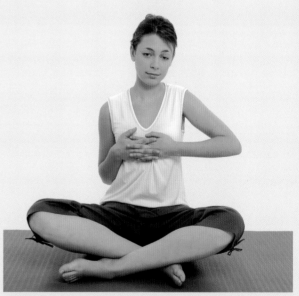

Centring the heart

The hands are clasped over the chest and the elbows are slapped against the body in order to help the heart chakra to align correctly.

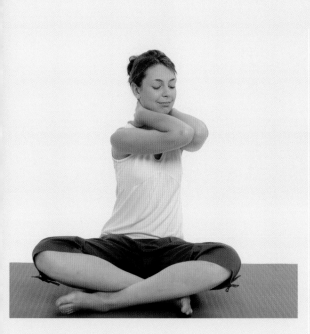

Aligning the chakras

The hands are clasped behind the neck and the elbows are brought together and moved from side to side to help all the channels and chakras to align and work together.

Opening the navel chakra

The hand are held palms together and the leg is kicked out, first one and then the other, in order to align the navel chakra.

Opening the base chakra

The hands are clasped palms towards the navel and the leg is spun in both directions, first one leg and then the other, in order to align the base chakra.

Opening the heart chakra

One arm is held by the side while the other is thrown out behind the practitioner in order to open the chest and the heart chakra. The movement is then performed on the other arm.

Profound spiritual practices

Tummo is the first in a series of profound practices known as the Six Yogas of Naropa that should not be attempted without a master. After accomplishing it, adepts can go on to explore the other five practices: illusory body, clear light, forceful projection, dream yoga and transference of consciousness at the time of death. By understanding such practices, we learn how the hidden force of the spirit is infinitely more powerful than a belief in the self, and that the intellect in the brain is not a reliable master.

Body-changing heat

The practice of *tummo* brings about a great, or 'wrathful', psychophysical heat in the body that dethrones *marigpa*, the delusory notion of an inherent self (see page 54). This causes a fundamental shift in perception – it blows apart the whole notion of self.

To achieve the state of *tummo*, Tibetan yogis focus on a syllable at the navel. As they practise in this way, the *rtsa* energy channels, *lung* and *tigle* drops free the life energy, or divine intelligence, *tsog-lung*, from the body. This ultimately generates the body of a Buddha. Such is the body heat created by *tummo* adepts doing this practice that, as part of a test of their accomplishment, they repeatedly dry sheets that have been dipped in iced water and wrapped around them.

'Since there is no deception, there is no fear'

Prajnaparamita Sutra

Secret practices

In the 17th century, the 5th Dalai Lama built the secret Lukhang Temple in the middle of a lake behind the Potala Palace as an offering to the *lu*, or earth spirits. *Lu* are guardians of both earthly and spiritual treasures. The temple walls are covered with murals that depict the Dzogchen teachings revealed by Pema Lingpa (1450–1521), known as the Realization of Vast Beneficence. On the top floor is the Sistine Chapel of Tibetan Buddhism: a 1.8 m (6 ft) square room whose roof is covered with murals depicting the path to enlightenment. Only the Dalai Lama and his close attendants were allowed to see and study the murals, such was (and is) their sacredness. They depict the hidden forces from which true spirituality is born. Contained in these murals are the secret Tantric practices, in particular the higher practice of Dzogchen, that are passed orally from master to close disciple. The northern wall of the chamber depicts yogic techniques for transforming the essences of the body into the light body of a Buddha.

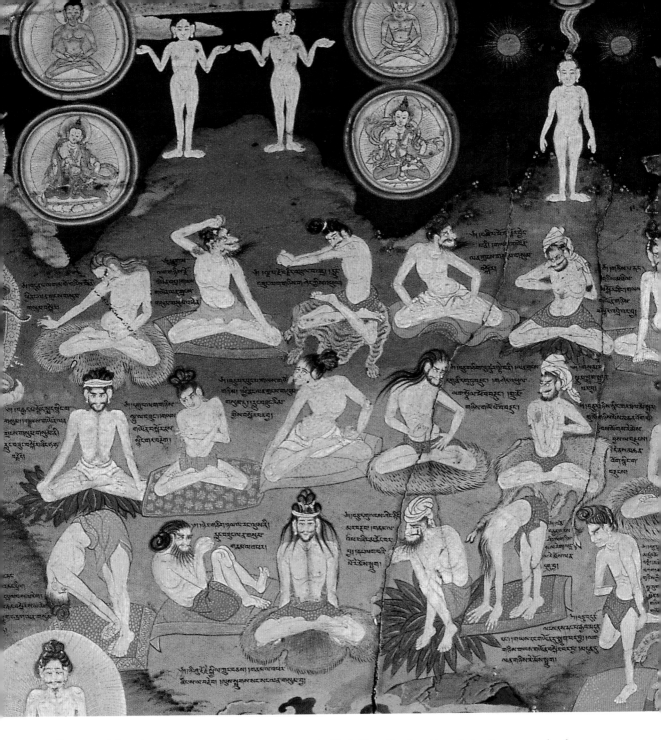

Researching *tummo*

This phenomenon, well known in Tibet, has for the past 20 years been studied by Harvard MD Herbert Benson, with the blessing of the Dalai Lama. Dr Benson and his team have discovered startling facts about *tummo* practitioners: they can raise their body temperature by 8.3°C (46.9°F) and lower their metabolism by up to 64 per cent. At the University of California, Dr Charles

The Lukhang Temple in Lhasa depicts the most sacred and esoteric practices of Tantric Buddhism.

Raison is studying *tummo* and depression. By monitoring its effects on the nervous and endocrine systems, he hopes to see what parts of those systems may be defective in patients with depression. Ultimately, the practice of *tummo* may reduce the need for medication in the West.

Healing dreams

Sleep is valued in both the Western and Tibetan medical traditions. To Tibetan doctors, sleep problems indicate a disorder of lung energy. In the West, lack of sleep is regarded as a symptom of stress-related illness, such as depression, and it is considered a precursor to ailments including neuro-degenerative disorders.

In Tibet, sleep is valued for the opportunity it affords the brain to come to a more perfect understanding of the nature of existence. In Western medicine, sleep characterized by its REM (rapid eye movements) is considered the brain's natural flush system. According to both systems, the best time for dreaming is between dawn and early morning – between 6 and 8 am, when REM is at its most potent, dreams are most lucid and the emotional healing aspects of the brain are most profound.

Life as a dream

Dreams help us make sense of the world and life, and so are significant in Tibetan culture as a form of mind-training. Tantric practitioners believe that if you are not aware in your dreams, you won't be aware of your daily behaviour. If you are not living consciously, you won't be aware of the direction that your life is taking.

By being conscious of dreaming during sleep, we can all come to understand that the waking state is just a dream, too. In fact, a dream is one of the metaphors used by the Buddha in the *Diamond Cutter Sutra* to explain the impermanence of all phenomenon:

> *'As stars, a fault of vision, as a lamp,*
> *A mock show, dewdrops, or a bubble,*
> *A dream, a lightning flash, or cloud,*
> *So should one view what is conditioned.'*

By being more awake in both states, we become more spacious in our interactions. Having the experience of illusory reality in sleep allows us to see how attached we are in the waking state, and so we can learn detachment by experiencing our dreams lucidly. Some practitioners become so awake in a dream that they are able to direct its outcome.

Tibetan dream yoga

In Tantric Buddhism, dreaming is a spiritual technology and makes up one of the Six Yogas of Naropa (see page 144). Yogis train their minds to have lucid dreams, in which one is awake and aware while dreaming. Adepts regard what comes from the unconscious in the form of dreams as more revealing than the conscious

---

Dreams in Tibetan remedies

A patient's dreams are taken into consideration at the beginning of treatment and may reveal whether the patient will recover. Auspicious dreams indicating longevity include deities, holy men and women, fire, safely crossing water or mountain passes and overcoming enemies. Dreams of death, corpses, falling and riding on animals are bad omens, even if the person is healthy. Tibetans who have bad dreams ask lamas to perform prayers for them and try to perform acts of generosity, such as releasing animals that are going to die, to increase their merit and improve their karma.

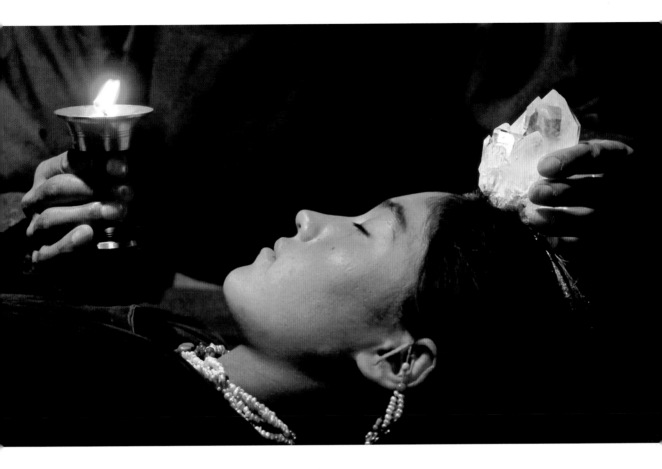

mind, and use the state to communicate with other realms. The more advanced practice of 'clear light' in sleep is a secret tradition, but the ultimate goal of dream yoga is to achieve recognition of the nature of mind, particularly at the time of death.

Many ancient cultures use ethnogenic (or psychedelic) plants shamanically as a tool to enter dream states or travel to 'other worlds' to expand their understanding of consciousness and the truth of how humankind distorts the true nature of reality. The experience has the potential to dismantle the egoic world view. Often the chemical DMT is found in ethnogens, such as ayahusca, and this 'spirit molecule' has also been found to occur naturally in the pineal gland, or third eye. It is heightened at spiritually charged moments, such as birth, death and when we enter mystical states, including enlightenment. Tibetan doctors would urge users not to get stuck on the psychedelic bridge, but rather to use

A Tibetan doctor places a quartz medicine stone that will clear the patient's mind and help her to sleep.

such substances to enter a bright world of everlasting openness or *shunyata*.

The healing power of dreams

Western science also values the healing power of dreams. For example, Dr Robert Stickgold and his colleagues at Harvard have a hypothesis that the REM during sleep metabolizes life events and reorganizes the brain. This type of REM causes a drop in heart rate and an increase in body temperature, and returns the body to a state of relaxation. So beneficial do these naturally healing eye movements seem to be that a therapy known as EMDR (eye movement desensitization and reprocessing) has been developed to process traumatic memories, or mental scars, in a matter of hours and thereby promote recovery from emotional suffering.

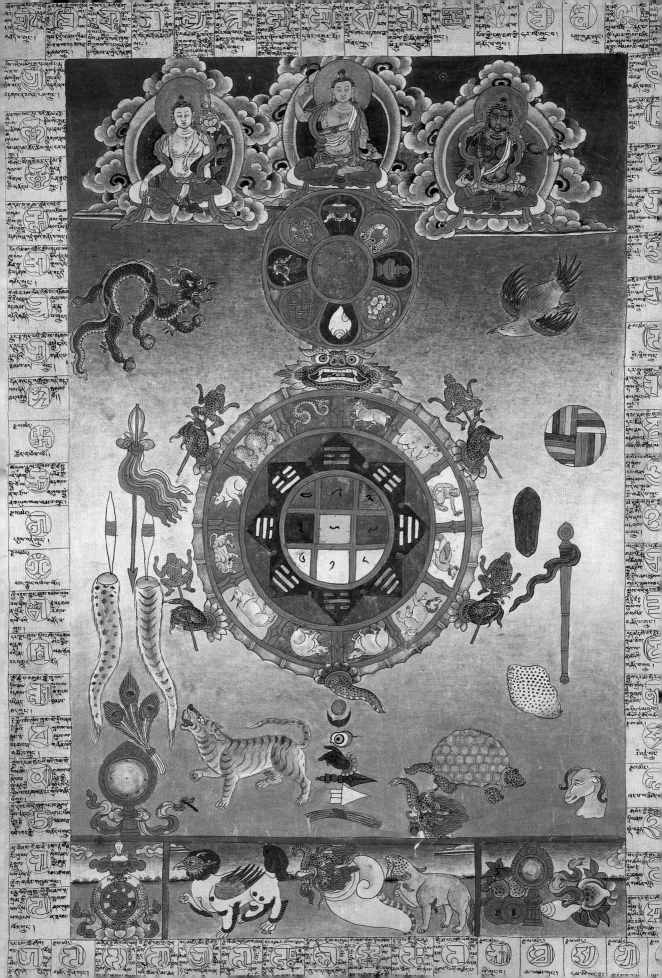

Psychiatric medicine

One of the richest subjects that the Gyud Zhi elucidates is psychiatry and the treatment of mental illness. For more than 1,000 years Tibetan medicine has helped those with mental-health problems through the use of herbs, nutrients and Tantric religious practices. This ancient medical system has therefore much to offer the West, which has suffered an epidemic of mental-health issues, such as anxiety and depression, during the last few decades.

Western medicine often attempts to deal with this problem through addictive prescription drugs. Worldwide sales of tranquillizers, sleeping pills, anti-depressants and other central nervous system drugs now account for an estimated $76 billion.

The source of mental illness

According to Tibetan Buddhism and Tibetan medicine, all suffering originates in the mind. Religion has always played a role in the description of mental illness, especially in shamanism, and the practice of *Dharma* for Tibetan Buddhists acts as preventive medicine for mental health. They believe that right view – selflessness or *rigpa* – and healthy moral psychology are both crucial for wellbeing and essential for Tantric practice.

All mental-health issues in Tibetan medicine are related to the vital energy *lung* and in particular to the life force *tsog-lung*. If the winds in the body try to enter the life-force vein *srog rtsa* at the heart, insanity will erupt, causing mental 'distortion', hallucinations or anxiety. Suppressing any of the internal *lung* energies, especially the emotions, also gives rise to mental imbalance as well as high blood pressure and cardiovascular disease.

Tibetan medicine, through its profound understanding of subtle anatomy, describes the heart as the seat of the mind. The *tantras* describe consciousness at the heart being made up of

'For Tibetan Buddhists, the practice of Dharma acts as preventive medicine for mental health'

This Tibetan astrological chart indicates the days on which a patient should guard against the power of demons.

three channels, five consciousness veins and the veins of the five senses. Mental illness comes about when blockages cause *lung* energies to circulate in the wrong direction around this physiological zone of consciousness.

Tibetan diagnosis

Tibetan medicine places mental illness into three categories: fear (paranoia), aggression and depression (withdrawal). They correspond to an imbalance in the vital energies *lung*, *tripa* and *bekan* respectively. According to the medical *tantras*, there are five causes of insanity: karma, grief-worry, humoral organic (diet), poison and evil spirits. Beginners of meditation can also come into difficulty as they release unconsciously suppressed emotions and undergo the terrifying experience of seeing that their self-aggrandizing ego is not real. This can give rise to an imbalance in *tsog-lung* and, in extreme cases, psychosis. Becoming aware that you are relating to the world from an intellectual position, rather than from the heart, leads to a drastic shift in the balance of internal energy as the airs of the channels that support consciousness start to move in different directions.

Inner demons

Five chapters in the *Gyud Zhi* are taken up with a description of diseases caused by spirits, three of which are specific to mental illness. These are not only the external demons that schizophrenics sometimes describe, or which the Christian Church seeks to exorcise, but the inner demons of self-clinging and the biggest demon of all: self-absorption.

Tantric Buddhism has a profound understanding of psychic energies in its huge pantheon of otherworldly beings, which includes Buddhas, *devas* (angels), *dakinis* and *dakas* (male and female embodiments of enlightened energy) and protectors. The medical *tantras* specify 1,080 malignant spirits called *gdon* divided into three types, with 360 demons in each category. 'Demons from ignorance' are spirits from above that cause epilepsy and can knock a patient unconscious. 'Demons from attachment' are spirits from below that cause skin diseases. 'Demons from hatred' are in-between spirits that cause depression and withdrawal behaviours. The fact that skin diseases are included in this section may seem strange. However, Tibetan medicine teaches that the mind is made up of subtle winds or airs that make contact with the outside environment at the skin.

The section on underworld spirits is the most esoteric description in the *Gyud Zhi*. It describes leprosy not only as a physical disease, but as a mental one. This may be understood as a description of psychologically ugly states of mind that people try to suppress and, by so doing, create a form of internal mental leprosy: denial, deception, manipulation, conceit and deceit. This poisoning to the enlightened mind within obscures *bodhicitta* or compassion.

Possession has physical signs and the Tibetan doctor can detect these through an irregular pulse and certain signs in the eyes or even marks on the skin. Urine analysis is used to determine which ground-owner demon, or *sadak*, is causing a disease.

Treating mental-health problems

In Tibetan medicine, dietary changes and herbal formulas are the first line of treatment for mental illness. Tantric practices and moxibustion are also performed with special prayers, and the golden needle technique (see page 118) is often employed. Relief from perceived demonic possession can be achieved by burning incense for protection or wearing protective amulets. *Sang* is the name for a smoke offering performed by burning aromatic woods and herbs. It is believed to satisfy the spirits so that they stop attacking the patient. One amulet of Manjushri (the deity of wisdom) is considered so powerful that it is said that wearing it can repel a bullet.

The deity Vajrakilaya is invoked to clear obstacles and subdue the forces that block the path to enlightenment.

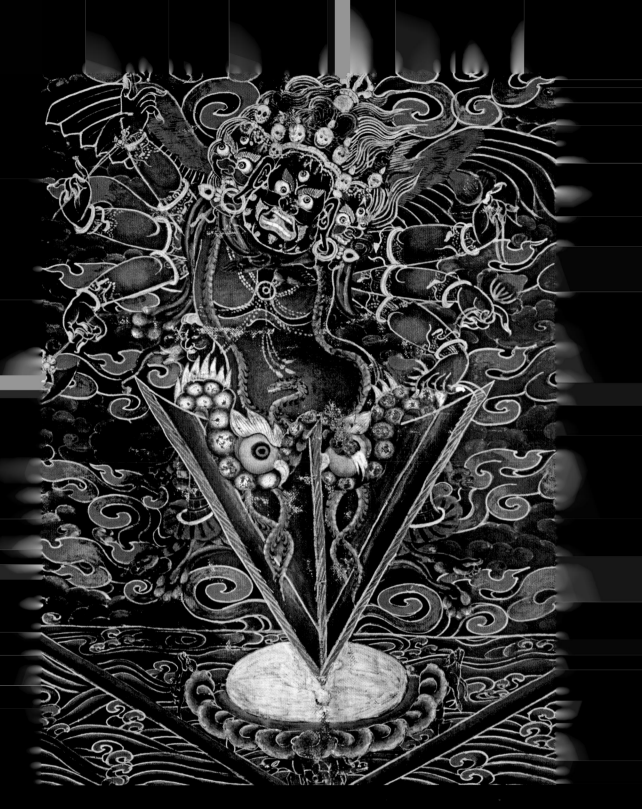

'A dagger that is so sharp it can pierce anything,
while at the same time nothing can pierce it.'

Dzongsar Khyentse Rinpoche on the practice of *Vajrakilaya*

Chod: facing your demons

Of all the Tantric practices performed by Tibetan Buddhists, the only one that originated in Tibet is chod. *The practice was revealed by a yogini called Machig Labdron (1055–1152), the most famous of many realized female Tantric adepts. She is believed to have been an emanation of Prajnaparamita, such was her interest and fascination in the* Prajnaparamita Sutra *(Perfection of Wisdom Sutra).*

How it works

Chod is one of the most profound and melodically haunting healing methods of Tibetan medicine. The practice helps to rid us of attachment to the thing we hold most dear – the body – and undermines our false notion of a concrete self. The goal of *chod* is to liberate the mind from fear into the great expanse of *mahamudra* (mind without objective). By cutting through duality in this way, one is believed to be able to antidote all demons, liberating them into cosmic space.

In *Machig Labdron and the Foundations of Chod*, Jerome Edou quotes the yogini's own description of the practice:

'Fortunate ones, keep this in your heart,
My instructions on chod
Are the authentic teaching of the mahamudra
This mahamudra *cannot be explained in words*
It can't be explained in words, but it is like this
Ma is the empty nature of the mind
Ha is the liberation from the vastness of samsara
Mu dra is their inseparable union.'

The practice in Tibet

Practitioners become fearless and perform this rite regularly at cemeteries, where the emotional energy of the self is intensified as the place scares or terrifies. Through practice they can become identity-less (neither attached nor averted) and

Beginning the *chod* path

Rather than running away or trying to suppress your own demons, such as anxiety, sit in meditation and face it calmly and with compassion. Ask it what it wants, and satisfy it by offering your body in the form of healing nectar. Through this practice, your mind becomes more and more peaceful. It experiences no hope or fear, it simply rests in nature of *alaya*, or supreme consciousness. A *chod* prayer session can take about half an hour, and during a *chod* retreat these sessions are scheduled four times per day.

give up a belief in an 'I'. Many great *chod* adepts in Tibet were, and are, wandering yogis. They summon all spirits by sounding a trumpet made from a human thigh bone. The practitioner's realization of emptiness, compassion and vast mental offerings (achieved by visualizing food, drink and nectar) dissipate the negative energies, thereby accumulating tremendous merit for the practitioner and becoming a medicine that heals all afflictions.

A chod *practitioner blows a trumpet made from a thigh bone to invoke the spirits and sever attachment.*

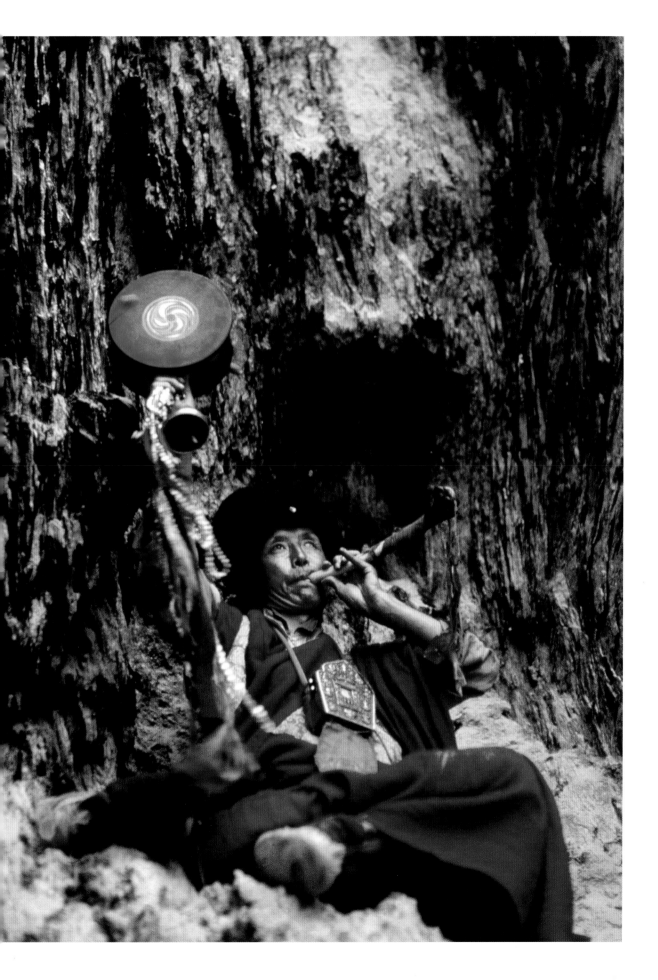

The supreme elixir of healing

Compassion is at the heart of Tibetan medicine and in particular bodhicitta —
the aspiration to attain enlightenment to liberate all beings from suffering.
Bodhicitta *is described as a wish-fulfilling magic jewel, since all happiness
comes from the realization of this expression of compassion and, without
bodhicitta,* Tantric practices are ineffective. Being of benefit to and loving
others is the very epicentre of enlightenment.

A Tantric practitioner always begins with the
pledge to practise in order to liberate all sentient
beings. Doctors of Tibetan medicine make such a
pledge, too, dedicating their healing work to the
enlightenment of all whom their healing touches.

What is compassion?
Enlightened love, as *bodhicitta* or compassion is
sometimes described, is explained in Buddhism
as being of two types: absolute and relative.
Absolute *bodhicitta* is the realization of one's
Buddha nature, a selfless state brought about
by a meditation practice that leads to the
understanding of *shunyata*, or openness. Relative
bodhicitta is the aspiration to attain enlightenment
to liberate all beings from suffering. This is seen
as a constant attitude in those who practise
Tibetan Buddhism.

The compassionate doctor
Tibetans say that if two doctors give medicine,
one with *bodhicitta* and the other without, the
medicine given with *bodhicitta* will effect a cure
even if its quality is not as good as the other
doctor's medicine. *Bodhicitta* is essential in the
practice of Tibetan medicine and is often the
quality that the patients describe about the
doctor who treats them. *Bodhicitta* is believed to
be alchemical in nature, transforming ordinary
actions. When it arises naturally, it enables a
doctor to know instinctively what is required to

*Tibetan medicine believes that a cure dispensed with
compassion will be the most effective.*

alleviate a patient's suffering. *Bodhicitta* equips a
doctor to make a diagnosis with discriminating
awareness and is thought to increase the healing
powers of the remedies he or she prescribes.
When the doctor uses his or her body and life to
practise *bodhicitta*, the incredible health and
understanding that follow may even allow
healing miracles to take place. The last teaching
of the *Explanatory Tantra* expounds that a Tibetan
doctor who practises medicine with compassion
will surely attain the state of Buddhahood.
Indeed, Tibetan doctors have been referred to as
'Emperors of Healing', for even a king must
listen to their health advice.

Putting it into action
One can mentally arouse *bodhicitta*, but what is
more important is actually experiencing the
feeling and expressing it. Understanding what
bodhicitta is conceptually is not the same as living
it. In order to put compassion into action and
achieve fruition from the practice, one uses the
six *paramitas* as guidance. These are: generosity,
discipline, patience, diligence, meditation and
wisdom. Everyday examples are giving food
and shelter; having a routine and life purpose;
enduring hardships without giving in to anger;
persevering with *Dharma* study; practising

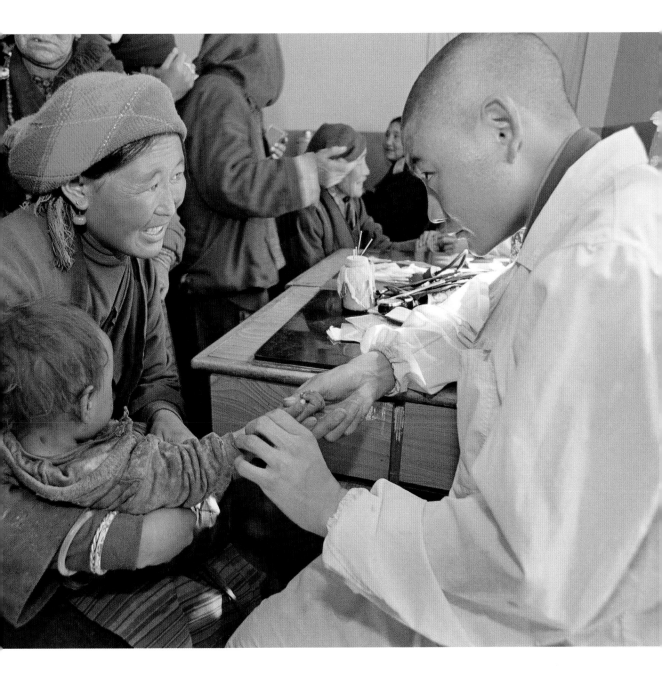

'Bodhicitta *is the powerful solution, the* atomic energy *that destroys the kingdom of attachment*'

Lama Yeshe

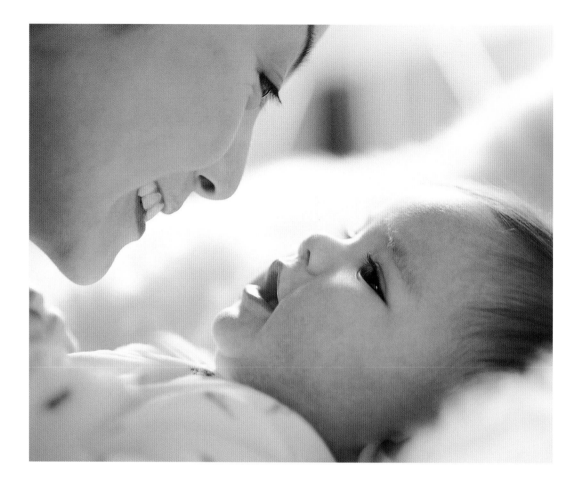

meditation; and understanding more and more the empty nature of all things. In this way *bodhicitta* becomes so strong – as strong as the legendary Mount Meru – that it never wavers, and merit follows. The merit accrued from the development of even an instant of *bodhicitta* is said to be as vast as space and to purify lifetimes of karma.

In *Vast as the Heavens, Deep as the Sea: Verses in Praise of Bodhicitta*, the 19-century guru Khunu Rinpoche describes the nature of *bodhicitta*:

'Bodhicitta *is the moon of the mind.*
Bodhicitta *is the sun of the mind.*
Bodhicitta *is the jewel of the mind.*
Bodhicitta *is the nectar of the mind.*'

Tonglen: exchanging self for other

One of the greatest healing methods one can learn is the practice of *tonglen* (see box). There

During the practice of tonglen, *you arouse compassion in your heart that is as strong as a mother's love for her child.*

are stories in Tibet of people who, when they were very sick and about to die, decided to give everything away and begin this practice. As a result they healed whatever needed to be healed within themselves, and without doubt brought benefits to those for whom they practised.

Tantric practitioners who do this practice become so compassionate that if a dog nearby is beaten, they may cry out in pain and suffer bruises on their own skin. Such is the depth of love that they develop. The practice is easy to do and can have positive effects for you, for those close to you and the wider world. *Tonglen* opens you up in a profound way so that you become a vehicle for universal healing, and by reducing self-clinging it becomes a doorway to freedom from *samsara*.

Performing *tonglen*

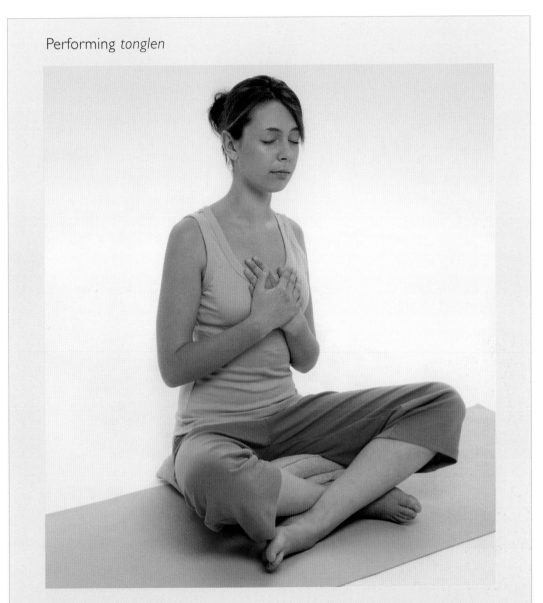

To perform *tonglen*, think of a scenario that arouses compassion in your heart and a spontaneous wish to alleviate suffering, such as a tragic situation from the news. Traditionally you would imagine yourself as a mother with no arms watching her baby fall into a river and float away. The feeling should be that intense. This is not a brain exercise; it must be felt in the heart so that contemplation of the scene gives rise to *bodhicitta*. Now visualize the person who has been most kind to you in your life. Imagine that person exhaling all suffering in the form of black smoke. Inhale that smoke of suffering into your chest, to the place where you feel the *bodhicitta*, and the suffering will transform into love and kindness. Imagine exhaling it as white smoke that is inhaled by the kindest person in your life. As that person inhales, witness them feeling better and their worries evaporating, leaving them in peace. Repeat the practice for yourself, then do it on behalf of other people.

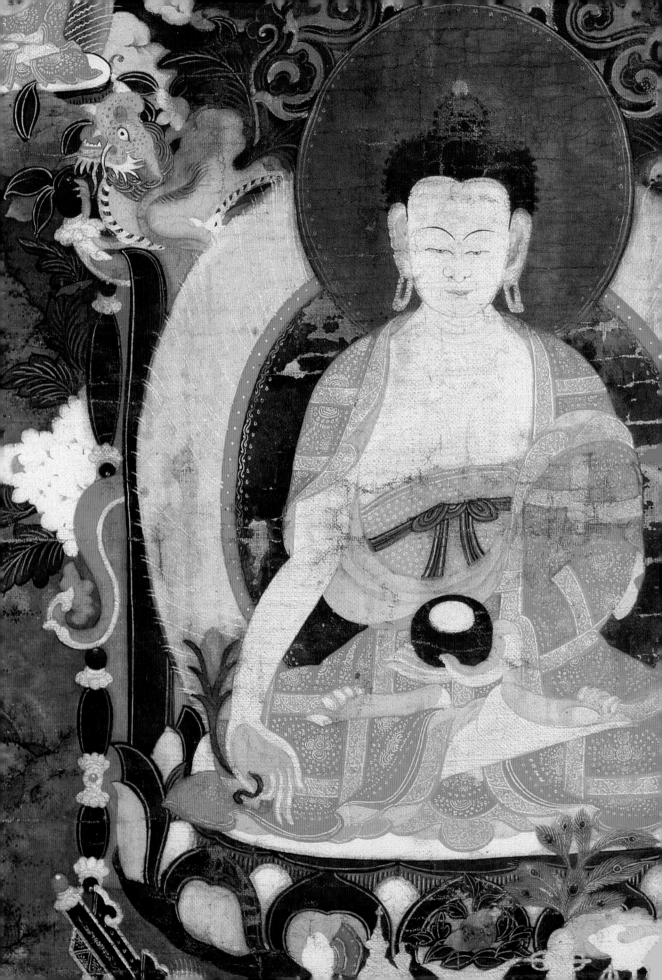

The liturgy of the Medicine Buddha

Everyone connected with Tibetan medicine prays in some way to the Medicine Buddha. Tibetan doctors perform Medicine Buddha practice daily — it is the first thing they do on waking and is repeated before they see patients. The practice is a way of connecting deeply with the healing energies on our planet and in our universe, and can help the devotee to develop healing powers. Traditional times for practice are the first quarter moon day (the Medicine Buddha sadhana day) and the eighth and 23rd days of the Tibetan month, considered auspicious days for healing.

Ritual in Tibetan medicine

People who practise Tantric Buddhism perform a daily ritual to a particular deity, known as a sadhana. For those practising Tibetan medicine, this deity is the Medicine Buddha. Each day, and especially before treating patients, a doctor will perform this sadhana, when he or she literally becomes the Medicine Buddha. There are 108 different deity sadhanas in the practice of Tibetan Buddhism, and each person is believed to have a karmic connection with the deity to whom they are drawn to pray and practise.

Traditional practices and vows

From the 8th to the 13th centuries, Tantric Buddhism flourished throughout India and Asia as far as Mongolia and Japan. Tantric masters (both male and female) are called *siddhas* and are best remembered through the lives of the 84 Mahasiddhas. From this Buddhist tradition, Padmasambhava or Guru Rinpoche (see page 26) became an initiate and then a master. He brought the richness of the *siddha* tradition of Buddhism to Tibet, to conserve and preserve it before the Muslim invasion in the 13th century.

As part of Tibetan Buddhism, deity practice (and especially the generation and completion stages) only occurs after the preliminary practices are accumulated: these are 100,000 each of prostrations, Vajrasattva recitations, mandala offerings and guru prayers. Prostrations prepare and purify the body, and unknot the channels. The mantra recitation of Vajrasattva cleanses all negative karma. Mandala offerings to your guru generate the merit that you will require to receive blessings. When you complete these practices you are seen to be properly prepared to be initiated into Vajrayana.

Most Tantric practices are extremely secret and are only given to close, trusted, mature and truly devoted disciples. They are normally performed nowadays in closed retreats in a monastic setting.

As part of an empowerment, which is an initiation into the practice by a lama, you may be required to make a commitment to do daily practice and take what are called *samayas* or vows. These *samayas* must never be broken, especially those between you and your guru. Whenever the *bodhisattva* vow is taken, it is said that a rain of flowers descends from heaven.

Daily practice

The daily practice of a deity is the epicentre of the life of a *tantrika* – one who practises *tantra*. Through the practices of the deity, the Tantric practitioner starts to identify with the nature of that deity. As a result of this, ordinary and supreme *siddhis* (accomplishments or spiritual powers) are realized. Ordinary *siddhis* are mind reading, premonitions, walking through stone like the great yogi Milarepa, the power to make mortality pills by transmuting mercury using alchemy, and an ability to find *Dharmic* treasures containing jewels and new teachings.

How the deity looks, the colour of the body, design of the crown, hand gestures and what it wears all have huge significance. In the practice of the Medicine Buddha, the deity holds the

Performing a sadhana (ritual) to a particular deity is a daily part of Tibetan Buddhist practice.

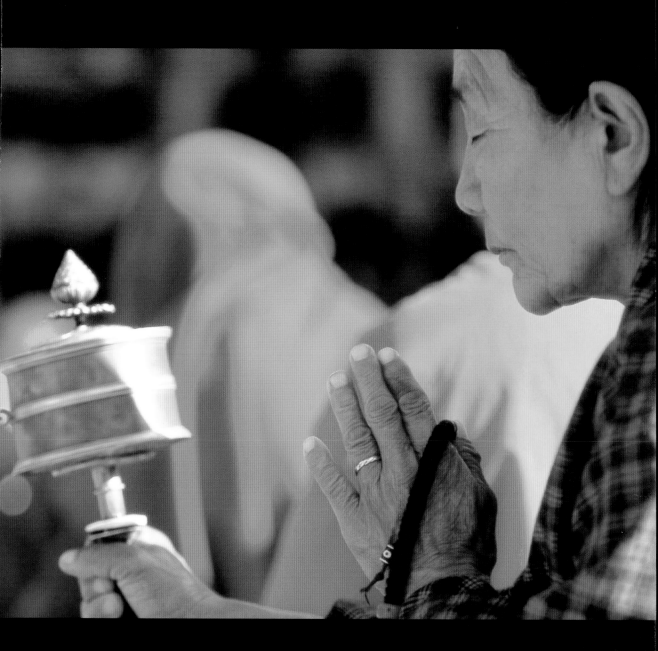

'Daily practice of a deity is at the epicentre of the life of a tantrika'

elixir of immortality in his left hand and a twig of the sacred myrolaban tree in his right, offering it to the world. His body is blue, to represent the sky as the nature of your enlightened mind; the colour blue is also cooling and pacifying. He sits in his healing paradise where everything can be used to promote health and wellbeing and eradicate disease.

Implements of Tibetan ritual

Tantric practitioners possess a bell, which symbolizes emptiness (*shunyata*), and a *dorje*, a ritual object that represents skilful means. The *damaru*, or small hand drum, symbolizes control over the body's subtle energies. The *kapala* is a traditional offering bowl containing rice that can be offered to Buddhas and *devas* (angels) as part of Tantric practice. The ritual described below (see box) is done as a prelude to meditation.

Using the Medicine Buddha *sadhana*

You can use the practice of the Medicine Buddha to help treat your own sickness by invoking his healing power. You can use it to bless your medicines (whether they are herbs or something else), just like a doctor of Tibetan medicine would. The liturgy can also be recited to help those who have just died, so that they may be protected by the Medicine Buddha and guarded by the *devas*, or angels, in his mandala as they travel through the 'Sidpa Bardo of becoming' – a 49-day state during which consciousness leaves

Tibetan ritual

Daily practice of a *sadhana* ritual will enable you to build a relationship with your *yidam*, or deity. It is also a useful precursor to meditation.

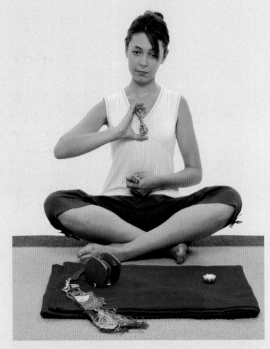

1 First centre yourself by holding the *dorje* to your heart chakra and the bell to your navel for a few minutes.

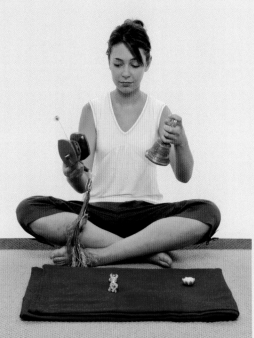

2 Then ring the bell and play the *damaru*. As you play these instruments simultaneously, you are energizing your subtle body.

the body and has many opportunities to gain enlightenment before undergoing rebirth.

The mantra of the Medicine Buddha is also very helpful to animals. Tibetan healing lamas believe that simply hearing his mantra is enough to cause an animal rebirth as a human. The practice can also be done on behalf of animals that are sick, as an act of compassion because they cannot perform the practice themselves.

Healing practitioners can use the liturgy of the Medicine Buddha to bless their treatment rooms so that they are imbued with his healing power. As a result of dedicated practice, you may even be blessed with paranormal abilities to help others. The Medicine Buddha ritual can also be employed to generate the success of projects,

and practice of the ritual is said to eliminate all pain and suffering.

Through regular contemplation of your deity and his or her universe, you start to identify with your own Buddha nature. Then, you may begin to act as a deity in the world, benefiting beings everywhere you go, rather than being stuck in the prison of egocentricity where you benefit nobody, including yourself.

One of the reasons that Buddha *Dharma* flourished in Asia was through the practice of Buddhist medicine. Through the practice of the Medicine Buddha *sadhana*, which benefits human beings wherever it is recited, Buddha *Dharma* may flourish again throughout the world.

The liturgy of the Medicine Buddha is offered on the following pages. As a *sutra*, it may be practised without an empowerment from a lama (see page 160). However, if you have taken refuge in the Buddha, you are strongly urged to get an empowerment if one is available to you.

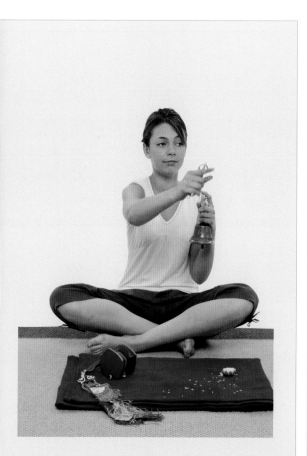

3 With the tips of your fingers, pick up some rice and throw it. As you do so, visualize the rice as an offering of diamonds made to the *yidam*.

Refuge and *bodhicitta*

By taking refuge in the Three Jewels – the Buddha, *Dharma* and *Sangha* – you can free yourself and other sentient beings from *samsara*; and by generating *bodhicitta*, your life will improve in all directions.

I go for refuge to the Buddha, *Dharma*
    and the Golden *Sangha* of Pure Lineage
Until enlightenment is bestowed upon
    me by
The Medicine Buddha and his healing
    mandala
By practising the four boundless
    qualities of love, compassion, joy
    and equanimity
So that all lower sentient beings and
    my children of previous lives
Who are lost in dualistic confusion
    and sickness
Be free from suffering.

May I be blessed with the grace waves
    of healing from the Medicine Buddha
    and bring all living beings to attain
    the enlightenment of Buddhahood.

Life is precious, difficult to gain, easy
    to lose and rare to find.
Death comes without warning as
    suddenly as blinking your eye.
Cause and effect cannot be escaped.
Egocentricity is the root of all
    suffering and disease.

Therefore I will turn my mind towards
    ultimate freedom:
The Medicine Buddha.

The seven-limbed prayer

Recite this prayer once, visualizing the Tantric lineage of lamas, deities and enlightened practitioners. This prayer purifies negativities and creates merit.

Reverently, I prostrate with my body,
    speech and mind;
I present clouds of every type of
    offering, actual and imagined;
I declare all my negative actions
    accumulated since beginningless
    time;
And rejoice in the merit of all holy and
    ordinary beings.
Please, remain until the end of
    cyclic existence
And turn the wheel of *Dharma* for
    living beings.
I dedicate my own merits and those of
    others to the great enlightenment.

Short mandala offering

Offering spectacular mandalas of the universe
to Buddhas and *bodhisattvas* gains a practitioner
merit and wisdom, without which no blessings
will occur.

This ground, anointed with perfume,
strewn with flowers,
Adorned with Mount Meru, four
continents, the sun and the moon:
I imagine this as a buddha-field and
offer it
[To the Medicine Buddha and his
healing retinue.]
May all living beings enjoy this pure
land!

Idam Guru Ratna Mandalakam Niryatayami

The mantra of purification

From the syllable *Hung* in this mantra, the
Medicine Buddha appears. Visualize him as
blue in colour and holding a vase of *amrita*
enlightenment nectar with his left hand and a
mryobalan plant with his right hand in the
bestowal *mudra* or hand gesture. He is wearing an
orange robe. The blue colour of his body cools
and pacifies all the 84,000 afflictive emotions.
Meditate that in the space in front of you the
Medicine Buddha appears in his healing pure-land
paradise, which is infused with rainbows. May his
eight related aspects cause a mighty rain of
blessings to heal all diseases that fall, grant all
wishes, remove obstacles and increase life force.

*Om Svabhava Shuddha Sarva Dharma
Svabhava Shuddho Ham*

Om – All phenomena lack inherent
existence – *Ham*

Everything becomes emptiness and
fantasy projections vanish into space.
Ah!

From this space awareness arises a blue
syllable – *Hung.*

The eight Medicine Buddhas

This prayer can be said at any time, especially around those who are sick, helping to purify and heal them of disease and bring about success in your life. Reciting the names of the Medicine Buddhas seven times, visualize them emitting healing nectars that purify all negative karmas, obscurations and disease.

1 Renowned Glorious King of Excellent Signs
2 King of Melodious Sound, Brilliant Radiance of Skill, Adorned with Jewels, Moon and Lotus
3 Stainless Excellent Gold, Great Jewel Who Accomplishes All Vows
4 Supreme Glory Free from Sorrow
5 Melodious Ocean of Proclaimed *Dharma*
6 Delightful King of Clear Knowing, Supreme Wisdom of an Ocean of *Dharma*
7 Healing Guru King of Lapis Light
8 Shakyamuni Buddha

Homage to the Medicine Buddha

By paying homage to the Medicine Buddha you are creating a karmic link with his healing mandala. This bond will grow over time and will heal not only you, but also the people around you, if you practise it regularly.

To the omniscient Healing Guru who
     is devoid of personality and persona
     I bow down and take refuge.
You are a Buddha in the palm of
     my hand.
You exist to remind me of selflessness.
You point the way to sanity and
     liberation from suffering.
One who has gone beyond fear never
     to return.
Who resides in a space of compassionate
     detachment from *samsara*.
Please bless me with your healing
     power.
Healer of outer, inner and secret
     sicknesses please bestow upon
     me the supreme accomplishment
     of selflessness.

Mantra of the Medicine Buddha

The sound of the Medicine Buddha mantra has a potent healing resonance and by chanting it you bless your body, mind and spirit as well as your immediate environment and all sentient beings in it. Through the dedication of the practice to the alleviation of universal suffering, you accrue vast merit and assuage diseases that have a karmic cause. Whisper this mantra into the ear of every animal you encounter, so that when the animals die they may be reborn in the paradise of the Medicine Buddha.

As you repeat the words, visualize healing blue lights being emitted in every direction of the universe, healing sick beings. Then visualize healing blue laser light waves being sent from the Medicine Buddha to your heart. Visualize this healing light filling your body and pushing disease, negative karma and painful memories out of your being.

Now visualize all sick and suffering beings cured and liberated as the healing light rays touch them. If you wish to bless medicines to make them more effective, visualize laser rays of healing light from the *hung* of the Medicine Buddha's heart, blessing them and increasing their effectiveness.

Dayata Om Beckanzai Beckanzai Maha Beckanzai Radza Samudgate Soha

Om — Eliminator of pain, healer of great pain, show the path of enlightenment — *Soha*

Four *Dharmas* of Gampopa

These four *Dharmas* describe the four stages of the path to enlightenment and bless the mind profoundly. Many masters have written books explaining the meaning of these statements.

Grant your blessings so that my mind
    may be one with the *Dharma*
Grant your blessings so that *Dharma*
    may progress along the path
Grant your blessings that the path may
    clarify confusion
Grant your blessings so that confusion
    may dawn as wisdom.

The heart of dependent arising mantra

This mantra is the essence of all the Buddha's teachings and is used to stabilize blessings and purify your practice. Through chanting the verse and reflecting on emptiness, obstacles are transformed into space.

Om, Ye Dharma Hetu Prabhava Hetun
    Teschan Tathagato Hey Vadat Teshan Cha
    Yo Nirodha Evam Vadi Maha Shramanah
    Ye, Soha!

Om – All things arise from a cause and it is this cause that has been shown by the Tathagata as well as the cessation of that cause. Do no non-virtue whatsoever, practise virtue thoroughly, completely tame your own mind. Such is the teaching of the Great Muni – *Soha*.

Mantra to increase merit by 100,000 times

By chanting this mantra at the end of your practice you are increasing its merit and its healing effectiveness, for the benefit of all sentient beings.

Chom Den De De Zhin Shek Pa Dra Chom Pa Yang Dak Pa Dzog Pa Sang Gye Nam Pa Nang Dze Oe Kyi Gyal Po La Chag Tsel Lo
[repeat three times]

Jang Chub Sem Pa Sem Pa Chen Po Kun Tu Zang Po La Chag Tsel Lo
[repeat three times]

Om Pentsa Driwa Awa Boghi Ne Soha
[repeat seven times]

Om Duru Duru Zaya Mukhe Soha
[repeat seven times]

Dedication

At the start of every day's treatment the *Amchi* or Tibetan doctor prays to the Medicine Buddha and his *devas* or angels in this way, to help him in the diagnosis and treatment of disease.

May all beings be free from suffering
May all beings be healed of disease
May healthy life-force vitality increase
May *bodhicitta* – enlightened love –
    spread continually as far as space
    exists
May earth spirits and their habitats be
    protected and honoured
May any being seeing the Medicine
    Buddha be drawn to chant his mantra
May all medicines be powerful and
    effect lasting cures
May wisdom and compassion grow
    and grow
May all beings evolve towards
    Mahamudra
May effective medicines be found to
    eradicate disease
May their side-effects be minimal
May the eighty thousand kinds of
    obstacle makers be pacified
May all mental illnesses be transformed
    through *bodhicitta*
May this world and the universe be
    transformed into the paradise of
The Medicine Buddha.
Soha!

Glossary

bekan Lubrication, one of the three vital forces of the body, located at the head.

bodhicitta The supreme elixir, compassion or enlightened love; *bodhi* means enlightened and *citta* means heart.

bodhisattva A compassionate person who seeks enlightenment for the liberation of others.

chakra Literally 'wheel', referring to one of seven energy centres in the body.

chod Practice in which the mind is liberated from fear and attachment by facing ones demons.

dakini An enlightened female deity who is referred to as a 'sky dancer'.

deva A Buddhist angel.

Dharma The path of truth, normally referred to as the teachings of the Buddha.

jalu The highest attainment of Dzogchen, whereby the practitioner attains a rainbow body by dissolving his body into rainbow light at the time of death.

karma The law that says for every action there is an equal and opposite reaction; cause and effect cannot be separated.

khor-lo The wheel of life; the Tibetan word for chakra.

kleshas Compulsive, afflictive emotions that poison and colour the mind.

la A specific internal life force that travels around the body according to the moon cycle, and is situated at the crown of the head at the full moon.

lama A qualified lineage teacher and spiritual friend; *la* means ultimate and *ma* means mother.

lung Winds, one of the three vital forces of the body, concerned with movement and located around the hip area.

mahamudra Mind without objective.

mandala A map of the energy fields in the universe.

marigpa A mind that believes in the self and is therefore deluded.

mudra Symbolic gestures of the hands and fingers.

nagas Earth spirits that look half-human and half-serpent, and which can bless a person with wealth, or cause disease if their dwelling place is interfered with or polluted.

nyepa One of the three vital life forces known as *lung*, *tripa* and *bekan*.

phra-bailus The subtle body.

rang-zhin The pure nature of reality.

rkyan ma The lunar channel, in which *bekan* energy predominates.

roma The solar channel, in which *tripa* energy predominates.

rtsa Channels that carry life energy around the body; there are 72,000 of them.

sadhana Daily ritual performed to a particular deity or *yidam*.

samadhi A meditative state or state of realization.

samayas Vows taken as part of an initiation into practice with a *lama*.

Sangha The practising community of Buddhists.

shamatha Calm abiding meditation, with which all meditation starts.

shunyata Emptiness-awareness.

siddha Someone who has attained supernatural abilities as a result of their practice.

siddhis Accomplishments or spiritual powers, gained as a result of practice.

skandhas The five aggregates of which the self is composed: form, feeling, perception, thought and consciousness.

sowa rigpa The science, art and philosophy of Tibetan healing medicine.

sutra A written teaching of the Buddha.

tantra A text containing secret mantras and visualizations, and the most precious of the Buddha's teachings, as it can enable you to attain enlightenment in one lifetime.

terton Reincarnate lama who is able to find secret tantras, called *terma*.

tigle Vital essences or drops that pervade the body.

tripa Heat, one of the three vital energies of the body, which is responsible for all biological processes and is located around the diaphragm.

tsog-lung Vital force, or the breath of life; it controls everything in the living organism and is driven by its karmic imprint towards rebirth.

tonglen Compassionate practice that gives rise to *bodhicitta*.

tummo Mystic heat; also a meditative practice whereby highly trained monks can increase their levels of body heat, drying sheets that have been placed in buckets of iced water and then wrapped around them.

uma The central channel, in which lung energy predominates.

vispassana A meditative practice that helps you to see things as they are.

yi zhang ma The subtle but profound consciousness located in the heart.

yidam Personal deity to whom the daily *sadhana* is performed.

Bibliography

Avedon, John, *The Buddha's Art of Healing*, Rizzoli International Publications, 1998

Bakan, Joel, *The Corporation: The pathological pursuit of profit and power*, Free Press, reprinted 2005

Baker, Ian, *The Dalai Lama's Secret Temple*, Thames and Hudson, 2000

Brazier, Caroline, *Buddhist Psychology*, Constable and Robinson, 2003

Clark, Dr Barry, *The Quintessence Tantras of Tibetan Medicine*, Snow Lion Publications, 1995

Clifford, Terry, *Tibetan Buddhist Medicine and Psychiatry: The diamond healing*, Wisdom Books, 1994

Crow, David, *In Search of the Medicine Buddha*, Tarcher, 2001

Dalai Lama, The, *Dzogchen: The heart essence of the great perfection*, Snow Lion Publications, 2nd edition 2004

Dhonden, Dr Yeshi, *Health Through Balance*, Snow Lion Publications, 1986

Dorje, Dr Pema, *Heal Your Spirit, Heal Yourself*, Duncan Baird Publishers/Watkins, 2006

Dorje, Lama Sherab, *Mahamudra Teachings of the Supreme Siddhas*, Snow Lion Publications, 1995

Drungtso, Dr Tsering Thakchoe, *Healing Power of Mantra: The wisdom of Tibetan healing science*, Drungtso Publications, 2006

Dunkenberger, Thomas, *Tibetan Healing Handbook: A practical manual for diagnosing, treating and healing with natural Tibetan medicine*, Lotus Press, 1999

Edou, Jerome, *Machig Labdron and the Foundations of Chod*, Snow Lion Publications, 1995

Evans-Wentz, W. Y., *Tibetan Yoga and Secret Doctrines*, Oxford University Press, 3rd edition 2000

Frazer, Peter, *The Aids Miasm*, Winter Press, 2002

Khyentse, Dzongsar Jamyang, *What Makes You Not a Buddhist*, Shambhala, 2006

Kunu Rinpoche, *Vast as the Heavens, Deep as the Sea: Verses in praise of bodhicitta*, Wisdom Publications, 1999

Leary, Timothy, *Your Brain is God*, Ronin Publishing, 2001

Lowen, Dr Alexander, *Bioenergetics*, Penguin, reissued 1994

Norbu, Namkhai, *Yantra Yoga: The Tibetan yoga of movement*, Snow Lion, 2003

Paine, Jeffery, *Re Enchantment*, W.W. Norton, 2004

Patrul Rinpoche, *The Words of My Perfect Teacher*, Altamira Press, 1998

Pearsall, Paul, *The Heart's Code*, Broadway, reprinted 1999

Perks, John Riley, *The Mahasiddha and His Idiot Servant*, Crazy Heart Publishers, 2006

Pinchbeck, Daniel, *2012: The return of Quetzalcoatl*, Tarcher, 2006

Rapgay, Lopsang, *The Tibetan Book of Healing*, Lotus Press, 2005

Rechung Rinpoche, *Tibetan Medicine*, The Wellcome Trust/University of California Press, new edition 1976

Reid, Daniel, *Tao of Health, Sex and Longevity: A modern, practical guide to the ancient way*, Fireside, 1989

Samel, Gerti, *Tibetan Medicine*, Little, Brown, 2002

Selzer, Richard, *Mortal Lessons: Notes on the art of surgery*, Harcourt, 1996

Servan-Schreiber, Dr David, *Healing Without Freud or Prozac*, Rodale International, new edition 2005

Simmer-Brown, Judith, *Dakini's Warm Breath: The feminine principle in Tibetan Buddhism*, Shambhala, new edition 2002

Trungpa, Chogyam, *Cutting Through Spiritual Materialism*, Shambhala, new edition 2002

Trungpa, Chogyam, *Glimpses of Abhi Dharma*, Shambhala, 2001

Wilcox, Joan Parisi, *Keepers of the Ancient Knowledge*, Vega, new edition 2002

Zohar, Danah, *Spiritual Intelligence*, Bloomsbury, new edition 2001

Zopa Rinpoche, Lama, *Lama Yeshe, Teachings from the Mani Retreat*, Wisdom Archive, 2001

For more information about Tibetan medicine, including contact details for doctors worldwide and online suppliers of Tibetan remedies, please visit the author's website www.stargatenutrition.com. For more about the preservation of Tibetan culture and Tibetan medicine, please visit www.medicinebuddhafoundation.org.

Index

Tantric yogis 56
tastes, Tibetan medicines 105
teas, herbal 89, 111
tertons (reincarnate lamas) 30
Theravada Buddhism 25
Three Jewels 164
throat chakra 57
Tibet 14, 26–8
The Tibetan Book of the Dead 41
Tibetan Buddhism *see* Buddhism
tigle essences 58–9, 136
tomatoes 91
tonglen 156–7
tongue diagnosis 13, 72–3
Trapa Ngonshe 30
treasure vases 63
tree of health and disease 45
tripa energy 10, 13, 15, 50
  causes of disease 12
  constitutional types 52–3
  diet and 93–4
  mystical channels 11
  pulse diagnosis 69
  and seasons 52
  tree of health and disease 45
  urine diagnosis 70
Tritsong Detsen, King 26, 28, 30
Trogawa Rinpoche, Ven. Dr 37
tsog-lung (vital force) 8, 42–3
  at conception 11
  and mental illness 149
  seasons and 97
  tummo and 144
tummo (mystic heat) 140, 144–5

U

urine diagnosis 13, 70–1

V

Vairochana 30, 140
Vedas 20
Vedic caste 20
vegetables 90–1, 115
vegetarianism 88
Vijay 26
vispassana meditation 128
visualization, chanting 114
vital force *see tsog-lung*
vitamin supplements 92

W

water: element 13, 52
  living water 60
  pollution 60–2
wealth vases 63
The Weapon of the Fearless One 26
West Malaya Mountain Six
    Excellent Medicines 106–8
wheatgerm 87
wheatgrass juice 89
wine 89
wisdom-eye chakra 56, 57

Y

yantra yoga 14, 140–3
Yeshe, Lama 15
yi zhang ma (profound
    consciousness) 12
yidam (personal deity) 163
Yidlas Skyes, Lord 22, 23
yoga 14, 138–43
  dream yoga 146–7
yogurt 88
Yuthog Yonton Gonpo 30, 31

Z

zodiac signs 78
Zopa, Lama 15

Acknowledgements

Author acknowledgements

Thanks to Rebecca Morgan for giving me a number of breaks in life, especially when she helped me to become a health writer, which has led to this book. Susan Mears, for being a great agent guiding and sometimes protecting authors like myself in the bardo of publishing. Jo Godfreywood, for having the vision to be the editor who commissioned this book. Ann Callaghan, for listening to all the ideas. Sandra Rigby, for making the book timeless. Fiona Robertson, who appeared in answer to prayers to excellently manage the book and steer it through edits, photoshoots and design with Leigh Jones to make it a success. Nicola Sweeny, may your spirit also benefit from the book. Fr Donal, for bringing the Gospels to life and being a true Anam Cara. Rosemary, Fr Francis, Georgia, Alberto, Leo, Aoife, Ross, Will, Maria and Kieran, Peter, Tsering, the McCarthys, John and Charlie. Lama Suzanne. Valerie, for always pushing me into emptiness, always standing by me and being my first kind Guru. And to my enemies too, who tried and failed to obstruct me.

Photographic acknowledgements

akg-images 8, 9. **Alamy**/Emily Wood 15; /EmmePi Asia 80; /Hemis 147; /imagebroker 85; /Sherab 52, 118. **AMNH: Anthropology Collection** 10, 44, 49, 51. **The Art Archive** 135, 158, 23, 24; /Musee Guimet Paris/Dagli Orti (A) 2.BananaStock 156. **By Courtesy of Dr Bhutti** 36. **Bridgeman Art Library**/India Office Library, London, Ann & Bury Peerless Picture Library 21; /National Museums of Scotland 18. **Corbis UK Ltd**/Alison Wright 5, 75; /Angelo Cavalli/zefa 11; /Christopher Bois 38; /Craig Lovell 62; /Macduff Everton 64; /Michele Falzone/JAI 61; /Reuters 34; /Roman Soumar 37; /Tizana and Gianni Baldizzone 103, 104. **Diane Barker** 67, 83, 100, 105. **Digitale Boekenstad Nederland** 71. **Frances Garrett**/Tibetan and Himalayan Digital Library 107. **Francis Apesteguy Photography** 123. **Fr.Francis V. Tiso**, Ph.D 31. **Getty Images** 17, 154. **Huntington Archive** 28. **IATTM – International Academy for Traditional Tibetan Medicine** 117. **Impact Photos** 55. **Mediscan** 119. **Octopus Publishing Group Limited**/Colin Bowling 92; /David Loftus 91; /Frank Adam 86 bottom left, 98 bottom right; /Gary Latham 97; /Ian Wallace 109; /Lis Parsons 93; /Mark Winwood 98 top; /Mike Good 1; /Mike Prior 136; /Sandra Lane 95; /Stephen Conroy 87, 88 bottom right; /William Lingwood 94. **Collection of Rubin Museum of Art** 27. **Science Photo Library** 42; /Alex Grey; /Peter Arnold INC 43. **Shambhala Archives**/Photo by Martin Janowitz. From the collection of the Shambhala Archives. Used by permission 129. **Shutterstock**/Baloncici 93 top. **Still Pictures** 151, 153, 161; /Galen Rowell 124; /sinopictures/READFOTO 12; /Thomas Kelly 73, 28. **Thomas Laird** 145. **Tibet Images** 32. **Vivian Kurz Shechen**/Matthieu Ricard 127. **The Wellcome Trust** 47, 59, 148; /Theresia Hofer 33. **Werner Forman Archive** 41, 77, 30; /Philip Goldman Collection, London 137.

Publisher acknowledgements

Every reasonable effort has been made to trace copyright holders of the following extracts. The publisher apologises for any errors or omissions and would be grateful if notified of any corrections that should be incorporated in future reprints or editions of this book.

pp.22 and 70: From *Tibetan Medicine* by Rechung Rinpoche, The Wellcome Trust/University of California Press, new edition 1976

p.42: From *Keepers of the Ancient Knowledge* by Joan Parisi Wilcox, Vega, new edition 2002

pp.66 and 67: From *Mortal Lessons* by Richard Selzer, Harcourt, 1996

p.83: From *Tao of Health, Sex and Longevity* by Daniel Reid, Fireside, 1989

p.106: From *Tibetan Buddhist Medicine and Psychiatry* by Terry Clifford, Wisdom Books, 1994

p.127: From *Cutting Through Spiritual Materialism* by Chögyam Trungpa, © 1973 by Chögyam Trungpa. Reprinted by arrangement with Shambhala Publications, Inc., www.shambhala.com.

p.130: From *The Dalai Lama's Secret Temple* by Ian Baker, Thames & Hudson, 2000

p.140: From *Yantra Yoga* by Namkhai Norbu, Snow Lion, 2003. Reprinted by arrangement with the Shang Shung Institute.

p.151: From 'Dzongsar Khyentse Rinpoche on the practice of Vajrakilaya' by Dzongsar Khyentse Rinpoche, www.siddharthasintent.org

p.152: from *Machig Labdron and the Foundations of Chod* by Jerome Edou, Snow Lion Publications, 1995, www.snowlionpub.com

p.155: From *Wisdom Energy 2*, page 63, by Lama Yeshe, Wisdom Publications, 1979

p.156: from *Vast as the Heavens, Deep as the Sea* by Kunu Rinpoche, Wisdom Publications, 1999

p.164: From *Essential Buddhist Prayers, Volume 1*, page 27. FPMT, 2006.

p.165: From *Essential Buddhist Prayers, Volume 1*, page 27. FMPT, 2006..

Executive editor Jo Godfreywood/Sandra Rigby
Project editor Fiona Robertson
Executive art editor Leigh Jones
Designer Miranda Harvey
Illustrators Cactus Design & Illustration Ltd
Picture research Sarah Hopper
Picture library Taura Riley
Senior production controller Simone Nauerth